# Praise for *The Zen of Helping*

"*The Zen of Helping* offers spiritual principles and practice wisdom in a profound yet delightfully readable manner. While grounded in Zen thought, concepts are presented in a framework accessible and acceptable to helping professionals from diverse spiritual traditions. Readers will find guidance for self-care as well as for effective practice in this deep and thoughtful book. This book makes a significant contribution to the literature on spirituality and counseling practice."

—Ann W. Nichols, PhD,
*Arizona State University,*
*School of Social Work*
*Director, Society for Spirituality*
*and Social Work*

"Through the gathering of wisdom of his teachers, the insights of his own clinical experience, and the deep spiritual exploration of his own personal journey, Dr. Bein has created a remarkable road map of 'pointing instructions' and guidance through the complexities of our hearts and minds for all of us in the healing professions. His book is a valuable tool for anyone engaged in the work of healing the suffering of others, and the work of healing the suffering of one's self."

—Larry Yang, LCSW,
*Guiding Dharma Teacher,*
*East Bay Meditation Center,*
*Oakland, California*

"I have read the book with great heart and joy. It is so well-written, original, clear, helpful, and wise. I think this book will be an invaluable contribution, not only to social work, but many other disciplines."

—Joan Halifax Roshi, PhD,
*Upaya Zen Center,*
*Santa Fe, New Mexico*

T0266812

# The ZEN OF HELPING

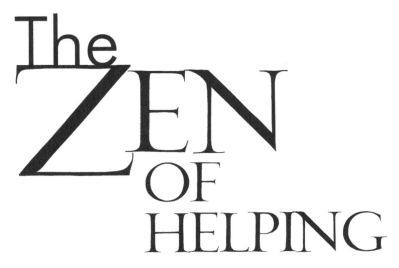

# The ZEN OF HELPING

## Spiritual Principles for Mindful and Open-Hearted Practice

# ANDREW BEIN

**WILEY**

John Wiley & Sons, Inc.

*Library of Congress Cataloging-in-Publication Data:*

Bein, Andrew.
    The zen of helping : spiritual principles for mindful and open-hearted practice/by Andrew Bein.
        p. cm.
    Includes bibliographical references and index.
    ISBN 978-0-470-33309-9 (pbk.)
    1. Counseling. 2. Counseling—Religious aspects—Zen Buddhism.
    3. Psychotherapy—Religious aspects—Zen Buddhism. I. Title.
    BF636.6.B45 2008
    158.3—dc22                                    2008008341

Printed in the United States of America.
SKY10086711_100224

# CONTENTS

# FOREWORD

Edward R. Canda, PhD

Professor Andrew Bein offers us an inside look at a compassionate, clear-minded, and creative approach to professional helping. He delves into his experiences as a clinical practitioner, a father, and a Zen meditation practitioner in order to bring out insights that are both personal and broadly applicable. His stories of what went well or not so well in his professional practice give authenticity, vividness, and real life sensibility to the recommendations. Students and seasoned practitioners will learn from this book through its challenges to rigid formulas and dichotomous thinking within social work and allied fields. His view is spacious enough to encompass evidence and artistry, strengths and adversities, planning and spontaneity, and ethical boundaries and boundless caring.

The word *Zen* is an English adaptation of the Japanese Buddhist term for meditation. Meditation can clear mental clutter to let us be vividly aware of the moment-to-moment nitty-gritty experience of our daily lives and our professional work. When we engage clients and ourselves in the situation with immediacy, clarity, connection, and openness, then genuine empathy and skillfully compassionate actions can flow within the helping relationship.

Professor Bein's approach to social work has been informed through Zen-based insights, but it is not limited to them. He presents Zen insights without the trappings of specific Zen traditions and religious beliefs. In this way, some Zen wisdom becomes applicable to professionals and clients who have no knowledge or interest in Zen per se. He has been open both about his appreciation for Zen and also about his intention to share insights without advocating for or against any particular religion. His studies under Zen teachers who have adapted East Asian–originated Zen teachings and practices to a worldwide context prepared him well for this task. For example, his teacher Joan Halifax Roshi, of the Upaya Zen Center in Santa Fe, New Mexico, is committed to socially engaged Buddhism that is open to everyone and that reaches out especially to the oppressed, the imprisoned, and the dying. This approach to socially engaged Buddhism is highly consistent with the professional mission and values of social work (see www.upaya.org/, retrieved January 3, 2008).

Dr. Bein's effort to extract Buddhist insights from a religion-specific context for wider nonsectarian use is akin to the development of dialectical behavior therapy, now widely used in mental health settings (especially regarding borderline personality disorder), which drew on basic insights of Zen meditation and philosophy as well as conventional cognitive-behavioral therapy, without explicit use of Zen terms (Hayes, Follette, & Linehan, 2004). Similarly, Japanese Morita and Naikan therapies have adapted Buddhist originated practices of meditation, self-reflection, retreat, and skillful action to a nonsectarian and spiritually attuned psychotherapy approach (see www.todoinstitute.org/morita.html, retrieved January 3, 2008). The psychiatric social worker Philip Martin (1999) has likewise looked into the way Zen can be applied in a nonsectarian manner to dealing with depression.

This book continues in a tradition of social work writers who draw on insights from existentialism, Taoism, and Zen to challenge prevalent types of interventions bound to rigid rules, roles, diagnoses, and prescriptions (e.g., Brandon, 2000; Krill, 1978, 1986, 1990). Such interventions are controlled, monitored, and intruded into clients' lives (albeit with good intentions) by experts who have convinced themselves that they know more than they really do. In contrast to expert interventionism, Professor Bein's mindful and openhearted style of practice has an affinity with the social work strengths perspective and positive psychology, which have shifted professional helping from a preoccupation with problems and pathologies to a celebration of aspirations and talents, surviving and thriving, solutions and recoveries, resources and transformations, and paradoxes and epiphanies of whole persons and their communities (Saleebey, 2006; Snyder & Lopez, 2007). We are invited into dialogue and partnership with clients.

As Professor Bein points out, this does not mean we should entirely throw out rules, roles, diagnoses, boundaries, plans, and evaluations. All of these can be useful within the context of a vital, dynamic, flexible, creative, and holistic helping relationship. As a Zen saying has it: being tied to concepts is like being a goat tied to a stick in the ground. Such a goat can roam only within a narrow range. Once all the grass is eaten, the goat will starve unless someone unties it. Concepts, theories, research evidence, and practiced skills should be in service to the real, emergent, and unpredictable particular happenings of the helping relationship. Practice wisdom uses these as skillful means for helping but is never tied down to them.

*The Zen of Helping* is a way of expressing spiritually sensitive practice (Canda & Furman, 1999). Spiritually sensitive practice is attuned to the highest goals, deepest meanings, and most practical requirements of clients. It seeks to nurture persons' full potentials through relationships based on respectful, empathic, knowledgeable, and skillful regard for their spiritual perspectives, whether religious or nonreligious. It promotes peace and justice for all people and all beings. We can be grateful that Professor Bein has shared his own spiritually sensitive practice wisdom in such an honest, accessible, and practical way.

# FOREWORD

Joan Halifax Roshi, PhD

This book is an important source of inspiration and wisdom for anyone in the profession of giving care, be they a social worker, a doctor or nurse, a chaplain, or a parent. Its contents reflect the values, skills, and attitudes that make caring possible in our relationally depleted world.

Some years ago, the author of this book, Andrew Bein, came to Upaya Zen Center in Santa Fe, New Mexico. I was moved at how he, a person of principles and sensitivity, absorbed the tenets of Zen, its practice, its very heart. He not only did so-called Zen practice, but he also attended the Los Alamos Bearing Witness Retreat that I had organized to mark the 60th Memorial of the bombing of Hiroshima and Nagasaki. Part of the retreat was at our Zen Center, where two Japanese survivors of the bombing gave powerful testimony to their experience. Part was at Los Alamos where we joined many others who were also acknowledging the truth of suffering that war engenders. There I think he really got a taste of what it was to "bear witness" as this was the theme of the retreat and we explored bearing witness from many different perspectives, and it was easy to get polarized in this particular situation.

In the many experiences that Andy has had at Upaya Zen Center and in his life as a father, husband, friend, teacher, and skilled social worker, he has crafted a set of principles or guidelines that make the work of harmonizing society truly humane. These principles are deeply embedded in the practice of Zen, which simply means to be nonseparate from all beings and things.

Andy says that Zen means to be intimate with all that is. This is what he means by authentic presence, a presence where there is no subject and no object, but where deep mutuality is present. This is the base of caregiving, of social work, of all human relationships, and truly of all relationships with all phenomena. We as humans so often need to be reminded that this kind of intimacy is no different than the right hand taking care of the left hand.

Andy also points out that the work of caring for others is based in what my teacher Bernie Glassman Roshi calls "not-knowing." How can we be with a client or a patient without the "diagnostic category" mediating our experience? Andy points out that the partner of not-knowing is uncertainty, and the interesting challenge of living in a world that is inherently characterized by uncertainty. But being a therapist or helper in a world of uncertainty might be difficult for some. Thus he suggests that we explore a way to relate to those for whom we give care with a base in the experience of immediacy.

Over the many years of teaching meditation practice, I have used the metaphor from the Tibetan teacher Chogyam Trungpa Rinpoche of "strong back, soft front." This has become a hallmark of my life because I, like Andy, often work with people who are caught in the terrible vise of suffering. If we look at the inverse of "strong back, soft front," we see that strong front is our defense against the world; soft back is our fear. So much of authentic Zen practice is getting this situation straightened out. How do we nourish the relationship between compassion (soft front) and equanimity (strong back)? How do we develop both tenderness and resilience as caregivers? This question is one that comes up again and again in my work with dying people, and certainly is important for anyone doing social work or providing counseling, support, or care.

Andy also values the development of mental stability and emotional balance so that we can trust our response to the world around us instead of being a tangled mass of reactivity and personalization. In this regard, he teaches us the wonder of the radical acceptance of the present moment, of what is, of things as they are. Only if we accept reality, all of it, are we in a position to transform it, and thus the theme of this book.

In this regard, our author addresses Glassman Roshi's second tenet after *not-knowing* and that is the tenet of *bearing witness*. How do we open ourselves to all the joy and suffering in the world? And furthermore, when we do respond, how can our actions skillfully contribute to *healing and reducing suffering*—Glassman's third tenet—rather than polarization.

In all this, a social worker or counselor must genuinely care, have empathy, be compassionate, and sustain presence in the face of suffering without collapsing under the weight of the pain in this world. Thus, a helping practitioner not only connects others to their own truth and to inner and outer resources, but as well connects himself or herself to inner and outer resources, and in this way practices good self-care.

The deep and wonderful work that social workers and other helping practitioners do is reflected in this book, in the real life stories, challenges, questions, and wisdom we find on every page. A social worker, counselor, psychologist, chaplain, or nurse is one who connects the visible and invisible dots through a deep practice based in caring, compassion, presence, and authenticity. This is engendered by loving attention to each being and thing, a fundamental practice of so-called nonduality in the small and great. This is the heart of Andy Bein's book, and the very heart of an authentic life.

# PREFACE

As helping practitioners negotiate and work within environments that increasingly objectify them as well as their clients, the demand for spiritual approaches to practice intensifies. *The Zen of Helping* is a pragmatic and self-caring guide that deals with the realities of practice. The book takes us beyond familiar and formulaic responses to client dilemmas. We develop specific skills that lead to our effectiveness with clients and we learn to view our interactions as sacred.

Regardless of spiritual orientation or religious background, your inner life is reflected on the pages of this book in a unique manner. You no longer have to be spiritually neutered while you explore how and why you work with clients. This book serves as a vehicle to discuss, understand, and accept your compassion and aspirations for clients, as well as your own disappointments and doubts. It helps you return to the essence of helping—embracing uncertainty and opening your heart—and to connect with the depth of your inner capacity to help.

This book is designed to be not only a vehicle for a validating heartfelt experience, but as a guide for you to tap into your own spiritual resources as you sit down with clients. Zen provides a foundation for enhancing your practice and self-care skills because its principles are congruent with the helping practices of social work, counseling, psychology, nursing, and medicine. You learn about the gift of practitioner presence and what it takes for you to give that gift to your clients. The book transcends or—as the chapter subtitles suggest—goes beyond traditional helping-professional books, which tend to admonish practitioners to be good nonjudgmental listeners, aware of counter-transference. *The Zen of Helping* deeply grapples with the real moment-to-moment issues for helping practitioners such as how to care while letting go, how much to consider the body and breath while maintaining presence, how to generate and maintain radical acceptance, how to create a container for client pain and trauma, how to be nondefensive in the midst of client anger, and how to cultivate courage and a sense of calling that influences day-to-day practice. Those with Christian, Muslim, Jewish, and eclectic backgrounds will find a home within this book. Each individual adapts the principles and practices to her or his spiritual or humanistic container.

I believe that the book's spiritual orientation and use of self-emphasis have profound consequences for practitioners and the clients whom they serve. The book will help the practitioner develop the proficiency to enter the uncertain world of the helping endeavor and create an environment where the client will thrive. Spiritual principles, thus, are pragmatically related to practice effectiveness throughout.

As one student with 4 years of social work training and a few years of field placement experience commented:

> The minute I began seeing clients, I let go of my motives and agendas, and just sat with them. The results have been remarkable. I can tell my clients appreciated being listened to, and really feel like they have a safe place when they are in session with me. I believe that is much more valuable than any theory I try to use with them. I had to let go of not being able to memorize all of the theories out there, trying to figure out which intervention I would use, and began to fully engage with my client at the present moment. This semester (second-year Master's student) is the first time I have ever felt that deep of a connection with any of my clients. I am extremely thankful for the opportunity to learn this skill.*

*The Zen of Helping* is not spiritual mush, however, where we learn how to hang out and just be present for clients. The book is informed by 23 years of practice experience that includes work in a wide variety of settings—from the Chicago and Sacramento public schools, to inner-city, Latino-focused agencies, to agencies with child protective services' contracts, to low-income substance abuse programs, to diverse counseling and private practice settings. Additionally, I mention some of my own personal struggles in order to make the principles accessible and to show practical self-care applications as well as personal successes and failures.

In Chapter 1, we learn that Zen involves being intimate with *what is*, and that entering a helping encounter becomes an opportunity to "awaken to the fundamental unity with the eternal universe right under our noses" (Austin, 1998, p. 12). The book is an "under-our-nose" guide that will enhance our practice effectiveness and our abilities to take care of ourselves. An opening quotation regarding Zen and helping is playfully

---

*Student comments are reprinted from assignments with their permission. Students were not asked to review this book.

analyzed. The chapter makes clear that the book's Zen principles are compatible with the world's spiritual and religious traditions. Zen is more about practices that align us with being awake, alive, psychologically healthy and intimate with the world, than it is about adopting a set of beliefs. The book's terrain is not linear, and you are invited to rejoice in the surprise, the paradox, and the ambiguity.

One of the book's main principles is discussed in Chapter 2—*strong back, soft front*. Zen teacher Joan Halifax has refined this practice principle through her years of service in prisons and hospice. Our strong back is needed to transcend the organism's fight-or-flight responses to distress or uncertainty and to provide the equanimity needed for a skillful response. Zen's emphasis on cultivating a still and settled mind is discussed here. Strong back metaphors related to the natural world and sitting posture—whether meditating or in-session—make the construct compelling and memorable. Our soft front works in tandem with our strong back. Soft front helping involves our open-hearted response to the suffering, challenges, and triumphs of our clients. Overall, the strong back, soft front metaphor leads us to move below our neck and embody the experience of helping.

Intimacy and practice with this concept profoundly affect the helping practitioner's outlook and practice. One skeptical student reported on the benefits of working with a strong back and soft front:

> Very helpful I must admit, and comforting for my clients. It gives them a framework of compassionate solidity from me and I think they like having that direction. It is like my yes means yes, and my no means no, and in the most gentle way.

The social context for offering strong back, soft front help is presented. Similar to the way kindergarten-through-12 public education objectifies children through test-score obsession, reductionist thinking is becoming more prevalent for people in the helping fields. *The Zen of Helping* joins voices with others critically examining the limitations of the evidence-based paradigm (e.g., Duncan, Miller, & Sparks, 2004), demanding that we face the nuanced reality of our work with clients, client situations, and service site contexts.

Chapter 3 discusses radical acceptance, which is one of the core principles of dialectical behavior therapy pioneer Marsha Linehan. Linehan's belief is that, by itself, cognitive behavior therapy's unrelenting focus on change is counterproductive and needs to be balanced with radical acceptance strategies and practitioner outlook. One student commented on how a radical acceptance thread was present for her:

> The nonjudgmental, kind atmosphere of acceptance in the class and the text has been liberating. . . . The ideas liberate you and your clients to be authentic and feel valued, imperfections and all.

Radical acceptance is not a stance of docility and inaction. It is argued that—through facing things as they are—radical acceptance prepares the practitioner to take constructive action. Radical acceptance is not for wimps.

Mindfulness is presented in Chapter 4. You do not have to be a meditator to teach or learn from this chapter. Accounts of practical mindfulness applications and simple exercises provide a glimpse of mindfulness' potential for helping practitioners. Guided mindfulness activities such as eating a raisin create memorable experiences that are generalizable to the practice world.

Although caring is mentioned often as a curative factor for clients, it receives scant attention in helping professional literature. Chapter 5 discusses the importance of caring and how we can manifest caring through our genuine curiosity regarding our clients' lives. Our waxing and waning energy to care for people is explored, and we learn how opening up to inspiration serves as a protective factor.

Bearing witness to trauma and pain is the topic of Chapter 6. Mainstream literature (e.g., Mollica, 2006) suggests that bearing witness sometimes offers the most powerful components in the treatment of trauma. We discuss how we bear witness to our own pain and how the boundless nature of pain and suffering provide opportunities to enter into a spiritual connection with our clients. The dilemma of maintaining client-practitioner boundaries as we sit in boundlessness is examined, and we consider the phenomenon of the "wounded healer." The wounded healer, as in the tradition of the shaman, may bring personal gifts and talents for bearing witness. Alternatively, the beginner's mind of the relatively unscathed may be perfectly suited. The chapter offers examples of each archetype. Bearing witness on the macro level is also investigated as a way to face social trauma and to respond effectively. A political action example is presented that is congruent with Zen's emerging tradition of socially engaged practice.

In Chapter 7, we explore how to move beyond a dualistic framework. In Zen, the middle way is advanced to illuminate so-called polarities that are actually two sides of the same coin—in other words, completely dependent on one another. When we embrace the middle way, we do not attach ourselves to either side of the coin, and thus move beyond dualities. We embrace the apparent contradiction between "no big deal"—one practitioner's mantra—and the need to pay careful, mindful attention to small details. We look at a common debate that occurs regarding the strengths perspective versus the disease model. My own experience having an adolescent daughter diagnosed with schizophrenia helps the discussion evolve beyond scholarly intellectualizations and dogma. Middle way applications move to a macro level, and the duality related to resisting versus surrendering to service site rules and structure is addressed. The practitioner who understands and embraces the middle way while working within institutional settings becomes an effective advocate as shown in a case example.

Throughout the book, we are encouraged to *let go of* concepts that interfere with direct experience. However, the description of the book's practice path is, ironically, laced with concepts. The very suggestion that our work as helpers is fundamentally about uncertainty is, in fact, a concept about our work. Ultimately, we realize that we embrace the middle way between being conceptual and nonconceptual and learn that the middle way itself is just one more concept. As Zen master Genpo Merzel (2003) says: "We are freed from this trap (of paradox) when we realize that there is no way to be free of it" (p. 133).

In Chapter 8, we develop skills for allowing our *client's* spiritual world to enter the room. We first realize the potential that the clients' spiritual views or religious practices have for transforming their lives. Although we may be uncertain how to proceed, we consider the possibility that it may be more unethical to not account for client spirituality than it is to ignore or gloss over these opportunities. We move beyond our fears and concerns and learn how to ask questions about topics like prayer or beliefs regarding a higher power. We examine the dualism between religion and spirituality. Some practitioners may have a degree of comfort with spiritual matters but much less so with religious practices or traditions. We learn to walk the middle way between religion and spirituality and start the conversation with whatever side of the equation makes sense to the client. Bobby Griffith's struggles as a gay adolescent growing up in a Christian fundamentalist home makes clear the reality of our need to "have the conversation" despite our different levels of knowledge regarding scripture. The conversation inevitably involves creating a dialog in an environment of respect and curiosity. This chapter may be read before others to provide a base for infusing "the conversation" into their work with clients or for conducting ethnographic interviews with nonclients.

Natalie Goldberg and Joan Halifax offer a Zen approach to failure. Failure does not imply being blameworthy, negligent, ignorant, or uncaring. In Chapter 9, we embrace the reality that things do not turn out the way we wish they would and that our efforts—however skillful or not—are part of the story or chain of events that involve client and/or practitioner disappointment, chaos, heartbreak, or broken dreams. Embracing failure means that we do not have to protect an image of the self. The way is paved to *forgive* ourselves as well as other people whose lives are similarly littered with failure.

This chapter offers personal life and practitioner examples of failure. As we acknowledge our own failures, we bring lightheartedness as well as soft vulnerability to our clients. Some clients have lost children to Child Protective Services because they cared more about drugs than about being a parent, some have destroyed their relationships through anger and violence, some have not known how to act in a given situation, and some have been in the wrong place at the wrong time. Our ability to embrace our own stories of failure allows for our clients to do the same (if this is what makes sense for them). Ironically, embracing these stories decreases their power over us.

In Chapter 10, we discuss our challenges in meeting the needs of our clients. Although we may shy away from the term *warrior*, it is important to face that we often need to swim upstream in order to realize the sacred path of helping others. As mentioned earlier in the book, there are those who seek to reduce the helping endeavor to quantitative puzzles and who may have little patience for the spiritual principles advanced here. In addition to swimming upstream against convention, we also meet our own medical, emotional, familial, and social challenges that test our resolve and our mettle. We therefore endeavor to cultivate the qualities that nourish the warrior's heart needed to negotiate difficult waters. At times, the warrior's path involves *letting go*.

The text of a Vietnam War veteran's moving speech illustrates the principles within this chapter. When we start with our traumas, insecurities, and failures, we let go of the armor that would prevent us from realizing the ultimate aim of Zen—to be aware and be intimate with *what is*. In spite of our difficulties, we realize our inherent fearlessness to love the universe.

The chapter concludes with a discussion about cultivating a *sense of purpose* regarding our work. How did I become a helping practitioner? What is this path I am traveling? How will my sense of the bigger picture be reflected in all of my interactions?

Case studies, exercises, anecdotes, and poetry make the book engaging and accessible. *The Zen of Helping* could supplement a practice text, particularly in an advanced practice or mental health class, and it could be a primary or supplementary text in a Social Work, Psychology/Counseling, and Spirituality class. Persons interested in the interface between Eastern thought or Buddhism and the human services or psychotherapy as well as those looking for spiritual sustenance in the helping fields—including nurses, doctors, hospice workers, community volunteers, public school educators, and complementary health-care providers—can embrace *The Zen of Helping*.

# ACKNOWLEDGMENTS

Thich Nhat Hanh would say that if you looked deeply at this book you would see the entire universe. I will only begin to touch on the numberless people who have offered me the love, support, inspiration, and teaching that have made this book possible. My parents were my first compassion teachers and the first people who showed me what "open-hearted" meant. My father's continued selflessness and care for my mother is deeply inspiring.

My wife Bella and children Emily and Sam have given me all the life lessons that anyone could ask for. I cannot begin to express what it means to live with the gifts of Bella's presence, Emily's courage, and Sam's integrity. I am eternally grateful for our family dance as we live the 10,000 joys and 10,000 sorrows together. Bella, thank you for always being there.

I have crossed paths with outstanding teachers to whom I am deeply indebted. In some instances, I was not able to provide a precise reference for their pearls of wisdom. Their words are part of me and may have entered my consciousness by way of a particular dharma talk, audiotape, book, video, or private conversation. I want to especially thank Zen teachers: Reb Anderson, Darlene Cohen, Ed Brown, and Genpo Merzel as well as Zen student and psychologist, Marsha Linehan. Zen Master Thich Nhat Hanh's books, tapes, retreats, and Community of Mindful Living introduced me to Buddhism. His heroic life of nonviolence and principled living reveals what is possible for humanity. I also want to acknowledge the profound teachings of Vipassana teachers Jack Kornfield and James Baraz.

Zen Priest, Joan Halifax Roshi's heart and wisdom splash through the entire book. Her profound eclectic insight, willingness to swim upstream, and commitment to relieve suffering are blessings for the world. On a personal level, I am grateful for her continued support, presence, and guidance. Thank you, Roshi, as well, for contributing the Foreword.

I want to thank Ed Canda, PhD, for contributing the other Foreword to the book and for his useful suggestions regarding the book's content. I wish to thank other professional colleagues and personal friends for their support as well as for their efforts to tune into the essence of the helping encounter: David Nylund, Dale Russell, Susan Taylor, Robin Kennedy, Jill Kelly,

Sylvester Bowie, Francis Yuen, Mimi Lewis, David Demetral, Sylvia Navari, Krishna Guadalupe, Santos Torres, Janice Gagerman, John Erlich, Ron Boltz, Lynn Cooper, Chrys Barranti, and Teiahsha Bankhead. Susan Orr is my ex-officio dharma teacher and dearest friend. I cannot express my gratitude for your presence, wisdom, and wonderful heart. Prominent among the many people who enrich my life are Kevin Smith, Paula and Miguel Barrios, Stephanie Brown, Noah Horowitz, Olivia Alvarado, Corina Delfin, Brenda Mitchell, Michael, Elizabeth, and Nancy Bein, Michelle Palomares, Roland Olson, Mary Reilly, Poshi Mikalson, and Reed Walker, who assisted with editing.

I am fortunate to have the support of two leaders who manifest a strong back and soft front, Robin Carter, DPA, Director of the Division of Social Work at Sacramento State, and Karen Larsen, MFT, Director of John H. Jones-Communicare. I also want to acknowledge Marilyn Hopkins, PhD, Dean of the College of Health and Human Services, and the Sacramento State University administration for supporting my moving forward on this endeavor. Lauren Evans, Adene Fordyce, Niki Otong, and Dale Threkel were part of a wonderful graduate class that was first exposed to portions of *The Zen of Helping*; thank you for your permission to use excerpts from your course papers.

A special thanks to Alan Rinzler at Wiley-Jossey Bass for his initial enthusiasm about this project and his helpful suggestions. Lisa Gebo at Wiley became the book's editor and then life interfered; her presence is missed as she is healing from illness. Lisa could write the book on mindful and open-hearted editing. Wiley's caring treatment of its employees makes me proud to be working with them. I also wish to express my gratitude to Sweta Gupta for shepherding this book into production.

Finally, I want to thank all the wonderful clients, students, clinicians, and helpers who have enriched my life. May this book—in some small way—honor your own truth, courage, and resilience, and may this book help others.

# Chapter One

# A SPIRITUAL HELPING FRAMEWORK FOR OUR CLIENTS AND OURSELVES

*Beyond Spiritual Neutrality*

> *Zen mind is not Zen mind. That is, if you are attached to Zen mind, then you have a problem, and your way is very narrow. Throwing away Zen mind is correct Zen mind. Only keep the question, "What is the best way of helping other people?"*
>
> —Seung Sahn

> *Not everything that counts can be counted. Not everything that can be counted counts.*
>
> —Albert Einstein

Zen is about being intimate with what is. As we enter helping relationships with real people, what could be more important? We offer them our authentic presence, our hearts, and our willingness to muck around in their pain and fear as well as in their successes and failures. As helping practitioners, we project the reality that we are on a sacred journey with our clients. We are profoundly fortunate to experience a connection with people in spite of the truth that we rarely *know* what we are doing. This vision of practice is simple but it is not easy to realize.

Conventional training in the helping fields increasingly reflects a different vision about helping, which we refer to here as a *story* about practice. Practitioners and scholars who are advocates of evidence-based practice, for example, like the elements of *this* following story quite a bit: (a) results from studies are enormously helpful in determining what to do with clients; (b) once we can reduce a client's complex reality into a more user-friendly diagnosis or problem statement we are better equipped to be helpful; (c) helping practitioners often are ignorant regarding the true value of research or they are too numbers-phobic, intuition-reliant, or irresponsible to base their work upon research findings.

Sometimes we use a fancy word for story and call it a paradigm. Nevertheless, no matter how much some people worship chi-squares and *t*-tests or believe in the importance of citing multitudes of prior scholars who have said similar things, it is the author's own story about the value of different helping orientations that determines the kind of human service or therapy book that is written.

This book represents a departure from most books and emphasizes principles that tell a different story about the essence of helping practice. These principles are rooted not only in Zen, but also in real-life case examples and personal anecdotes that illustrate the principles' meaning, relevance, and application. At the end of this chapter, I make some suggestions on how to engage with this book. The book's core practice principles are outlined next, followed by a discussion connecting helping practice with practitioner self-care:

### Spiritual Principles of Helping

- The main ground of helping and professional practice is uncertainty and not knowing. Although theory and knowledge of the other may be helpful, it often interferes with our direct perception and engagement with clients.
- We are best able to serve our clients if our hearts remain open to them, we act in a compassionate manner, and we love them. The Zen metaphor "strong back, soft front" reminds us that our work also involves the area below our neck, and that our open-heartedness flourishes when we are stable and clear and the relationship has structure.
- We view our encounters with clients as personal opportunities for being alive and fully present in the moment. Our moment-to-moment self-awareness and presence is a precious and vital asset for clients.

Self-awareness is not about self-obsession regarding performance; thus, we are not distracted while we pay attention to the world of self and other. Effectiveness with clients and practitioner self-care are interrelated.

- As we increasingly trust the present moment, our responses emerge from deep wisdom rather than fight-or-flight reactions or superficial attempts at grasping for certainty.
- Radical acceptance of *what is*—in the form of our clients' lives, agency, or community conditions as well as our own responses, moods, or thoughts—provides a base of *transformation and change*. Although the term may seem to imply otherwise, radical acceptance is not about rolling over in the face of oppression.
- Bearing witness is the manner in which we deal with our clients' trauma and our own trauma. It involves our willingness to enter uncertainty and listen deeply, our nonattachment to outcome, and our ability to hold the client's pain without being overwhelmed. Bearing witness to social realities provides a foundation for engaging and acting with communities.
- We are *intimately connected* with our clients and communities. We tune into our essential nonseparateness in a manner that is spiritual. This nonseparateness means that my client's narrative is my own and were it not for some circumstances or biological or social conditions, I could easily be in the client's chair, and she could be in mine. We fully embrace that we, as practitioners, are no better than our clients.
- We see through the limited thinking that portrays many issues as dualities. The Middle Way allows us to simultaneously embrace *DSM* concepts and the strengths perspective without being attached to either one. (No *DSM* axe to grind here; I have two *DSM*-labeled children.) We are playful amidst the paradox of our nonseparateness or boundlessness with clients on the one hand, and the boundaries that we operate from in the relative world on the other. We do not contrive intellectual arguments that demonize one apparent polarity while extolling the virtues of the other (except for my few jabs at evidence-based practice).
- Caring for clients is rarely talked about in social work, counseling, and psychology, yet clients consistently identify practitioner caring as a curative factor. We focus on the nature and depth of our caring, which involves our genuine curiosity regarding who our clients are and how they live. As we move through diverse environments, we let our clients teach us valuable life lessons and inspire us through their courage and perseverance. We enter these environments with few preconceptions and a love of the unknown.

- We persistently take risks. We develop mindfulness regarding our fears or periods of low energy and witness them with detachment. We act with a warrior's commitment to the truth and to being genuinely helpful. As we risk and advocate, we are mindful of fostering peaceful, collaborative relationships using "right speech." We develop the courage to confront and to examine our own armor.
- We focus on our own mental, spiritual, and physical health. We embrace our failures and recognize that failure is inevitable within our lives and in our work with clients. Our joy, calmness, and authenticity are precious resources for our clients. We maintain equanimity while we are with clients and while we are away from clients.
- We use our breath to nourish our strong back and soft front. We stay centered and do not become attached or overly enamored with any story about the nature of helping practice—*including this story!*

## SPIRITUAL PRACTICE AND SELF-CARE

As we learn, practice, and embody the principles found throughout the book, we tap into previously underutilized personal resources in the service of our clients. We notice that we are less distracted during our sessions. We start to listen to clients with our hearts as well as our heads and our responses emerge less from flight-or-fight reactions, judgments, and dispassionate, label-based interventions. We begin to allow ourselves to care about our clients, to be inspired by their stories, and come face to face with their pain and the reality that we mutually toil in the unknown.

We proceed in this exploration grounded in Zen thought that emphasizes "each moment's sacramental quality" (Austin, 1998, p. 12). Thus, we do everything that we can in order to come into each moment fully. We increasingly experience sitting down with a client, family, or group as a sacred event that we are most fortunate to be part of. Our presence is founded on our radical acceptance of the feelings, thoughts, and circumstances that arise in our lives, our clients' lives, and the moment-to-moment experience that unfolds as we sit together.

This journey is a spiritual one in that it calls on us to go beyond what is apparent or what can easily be reduced and described in a book. The particular flavor of this journey in Zen is often simple. Our calm, open-hearted, sincere, and mindful approach while engaging with or attending to the smallest act allows us to touch the deepest level of truth—what some may label as the divine or God. As a metaphor, we notice that atomic and subatomic structures have the same patterns of orbit, movement, space, and unpredictability as the cosmos. As we perceive the reality of atoms, molecules, and quarks, we perceive the reality of stars, planets, and the universe. In a similar manner, our mindful, compassionate connection with one client in an office links us with all human beings in the world.

It is no small act, then, to enter a helping encounter for it becomes our opportunity to "awaken to the fundamental unity with that eternal universe, right under our noses" (Austin, 1998, p. 12). This book will serve as your under-the-nose guide.

Under your nose, just within an office or client living room is the client-practitioner gestalt right in the middle of the universe. How do you bring yourself to this encounter? How do you work with what is really happening— including everything that is happening within you? How do you cultivate the deepest levels of acceptance for your client and what do you do when serious judgments arise? What is deep listening and stillness? Are they "things" you admonish yourself to do? What role do your breath and posture play? How do you confront when you care and how do you make use of diagnostic labels when you want to transcend them? What happens when your own energy is low, when you experience failure, or you come face-to-face with difficult trauma? What is the reason you are doing this work and how do you manifest your sense of calling or purpose in your day-to-day interactions with clients and colleagues?

We grapple with these questions in order to provide the best possible service for our clients and we commit to a spiritual orientation because we understand that our clients need more from us than technique- or diagnosis-driven approaches. Although relationship factors are at least twice as important in determining outcomes as intervention choice or counseling technique (Duncan, Miller, & Sparks, 2004), conventional helping paradigms view the relationship as setting the table for doing the real work—assessing the client and settling on an intervention. In social work education, for example, this emphasis is manifested through the worshipping of the biopsychosocial assignment. Students, sometimes during three separate levels of practice classes— Bachelor's, first year Master's and second year Master's—write long assessments regarding the biological, psychological, and social or ecological factors that may have some bearing on their clients' lives. Once the biopsychosocial Holy Grail is complete, a plan for intervention is written that is often only remotely connected to all the information gathering that came before it.

Typically, little if any student self-reflection occurs around the spiritually oriented questions posed earlier. What judgments arise while in the presence of the client? How distracted or present is the student helper? How much has a sense of caring been cultivated in the course of the relationship? In what manner has the client inspired the student and has the student been able to communicate this? The biopsychosocial exercise reinforces the notion that we the practitioners "work on" the clients in a similar manner that an auto mechanic works on a car. With the interjection of the concept of counter-transference, we do acknowledge that we may bring some of our own dirty baggage (or dirty car parts) to the encounter that requires us to proceed with caution. However, we lack depth in investigating how our internal life can make a profound difference for our clients.

The spiritual principles in this book address the practitioner's internal life. Although they were developed with the "eyes on the prize"—practitioner effectiveness with clients—they inevitably address practitioner health and self-care. One group of students who were guinea pigs for much of the book's content commented that experiencing, investigating, and learning about *self-care* was a major outcome. Although not framed specifically in this manner, the book's emphasis on: (a) awareness of internal life; (b) use of breath to facilitate calmness and mindfulness presence; (c) cultivation of radical acceptance of self, other, and context; (d) celebrating the capacity for caring for others and, in general, invoking our heart within our work; (e) appreciating the balance between a strong back (container and structure for work) and soft front (compassionate heart); (f) facing trauma and difficulty without the customary and sometimes unhelpful responses of denial; and (g) maintaining a warrior's mentality blazed a trail for practitioner self-compassion, self-awareness, and self-care.

This trail was uniquely connected to practitioner practice—as one might expect in Zen. There were some discussions about self-care in the form of personal retreat time and mindful breathing exercises, but much of it was oriented toward integrating self-care with the in-session work with clients.

## UNIVERSAL APPLICATION FOR ALL TRADITIONS

People from many religious backgrounds, traditions, and degrees of formality as well as varying levels of faith or belief in God (from 0 to 100) found a home within these pages. The principles presented within are pragmatic rather than dogmatic and readers are able to apply their sense of spirituality to the concepts in the book. For example, a field of radical acceptance for some people is read as a field of Jesus' love. Zen's emphasis on encounters and interactions as sacred and linked to the "bigger picture" is similar to the slogan "what would Jesus do" for waking us up to the importance of our acts. People from Jewish, Shamanic, Muslim, and secular humanist roots embrace the book's specific lessons and orientation. A brief introduction to Buddhism and Zen can be found in the Appendix.

## HOW TO ENGAGE WITH THIS BOOK

"Zen mind is not Zen mind" was the first sentence of the opening quote. What a ridiculous and truly delightful thing to say. The idea here is not to try to grab onto what Zen is. Tightly holding onto a view or concept interferes with our ability to connect with the world as it is.

You are not asked to let go of any spiritual practices or religious views that you have. Zen thought is compatible with the world's spiritual and religious traditions. Zen is more about practices that align us with being awake, alive, psychologically healthy, and intimate with the world than it is about adopting a set of beliefs. If something in this book does not work for you, throw it out with glee.

"Throwing away Zen mind is correct Zen mind" is another sentence within the quote. The Zen tradition is full of playful paradoxes. On the one hand, the playfulness suggests we not take it too seriously, especially when we are exhorted to throw away our notions about Zen. On the other hand, the message within may be quite profound. We learn to hold both sides of this paradox—a lesson that has profound practice implications, as we will see in Chapter 7.

This book is a call to the heart and, ultimately, to the real world of practice. Examples are drawn from my experiences with highly diverse practitioners and clients who have been mandated, semi-voluntary, or voluntary. Because the principles are fluid, they will come alive as you become intimate with the book's content. A beginner's mind (Suzuki, 1970) is valuable. Too much confidence about material within may interfere with needed humility and make you think that you know more than you actually do.

Finally, the process of opening your heart to the book is parallel to opening your heart with your clients. The terrain is not linear and we are invited to rejoice in the surprise, the paradox, and the ambiguity. Just as we sometimes learn powerful lessons from watching a movie, reading a novel, or listening to a poem, the attempt here is to engage you in a nonconventional way. I wish to warn you, however, that explorations regarding practitioner presence, open-heartedness, nondualistic thinking, and client-practitioner connectedness are sometimes viewed as "nonprofessional." You may decide that it is safer to read this book in the privacy of your own home.

*Enjoy the ride!*

# Chapter Two

# SITTING WITH CLIENTS ON UNCERTAIN GROUND: STRONG BACK, SOFT FRONT

*Beyond Evidence-Based Practice*

> *Allow it all to be,*
> *no need to grasp or push away.*
> *Present with each moment,*
> *the whole of you, body, mind*
> *and soul, opens to receive.*

—Danna Faulds

This book is a little different from most social work, counseling, or psychotherapy books because it begins with the premise that we do not truly *know* who our client is or what we are doing when we engage in practice. No matter how many books we have read, no matter how many similar clients we have seen, no matter how much we think that we can relate to the client's life, no matter how closely we have listened to "the problem," no matter how many standardized instruments we have utilized, our story about the client sitting across from us, to a large extent, represents our projections or fantasies. We can categorize the client according to his or her race/ethnicity, mental illness diagnosis, presenting problems, strengths, substance use, behavioral transgressions, or milestone events or traumas; yet the environment of practitioner uncertainty and not-knowing most fundamentally characterizes the nature of our work with clients.

We learn to embrace uncertainty and not knowing and actually make this reality work for us. We look outside the professional helper paradigms that say that practice is about connecting the dots between the characteristics of the other (assessment of the client) and our bag of tricks (clinical or meso/macro interventions). In fact, traditional psychology, social work, and counseling practice texts and scholarship largely ignore the practitioner's inner life, process, or transformation. Read the slew of recent books on working with one form or another of mental illness, behavioral problem, or sexual orientation, and you will hardly find a trace of the practitioner. Somehow the practitioner's presence, ability to deal with ambiguity, energy level, fear, despair, compassion, or love is hardly consequential in the equation related to client betterment. The unstated implication is that the practitioner is a spiritually and emotionally neutered empty box who processes information and sits on guard against counter-transference or class/race or religious value judgments that would contaminate the otherwise elegant connection between assessment and intervention.

The notion of strong back, soft front grapples with the delightful questions related to what goes on inside the box—ourselves as practitioners—and how our vision, open-heartedness, awareness, authenticity, presence, groundedness, curiosity, and clarity contribute to mutually transformative client-practitioner relationships. As we conduct this investigation, we realize that the Western-oriented duality concerning client or patient on the one hand and helping practitioner on the other melts away and is replaced with a vision—grounded in Zen thought—of the client-practitioner relationship being one of interdependence and opportunity for mutual awakening.

Other dualities that confuse us and limit our potential for mutually transformative practice will be examined in Chapter 7. We consider the importance of time-honored practices related to practitioner boundaries even while we discuss the nature of boundlessness; we embrace the utility of categorical thinking even while we come to an understanding of the nonessential nature of our profession's social constructions.

## STRONG BACK

In the midst of all this analysis, there are few certainties to hang on to. We need a strong back to navigate this field of investigation and to enter into deep, transformative relationships with clients. Zen teacher and priest, hospice worker, health worker trainer, prison group leader, activist, and anthropologist, Joan Halifax, PhD, states that a strong back is needed so that the practitioner maintains equanimity in the face of turmoil, confusion, suffering, and despair. The strong back, as emphasized in Zen meditation, is the stable posture that serves as the sky for any storm clouds that are passing through; it is a metaphor for the never-ending calm breath that can hold the world's suffering and pain. The strong back allows us to transcend our organism's programmed flight-or-fight response to distress and provides the foundation of equanimity needed for a skillful response. Even in the midst of dramatic rainfall, rushing rivers, mud slides, drought, wind, fire, and plant and animal cycles of life and death, mountains—the ultimate strong back metaphor—hold all of this spectacular drama with solidity. In a way, mountains are nothing more than a conglomeration of all of these elements and dynamics, and thus represent home for them. As the rivers of emotions and thoughts flow through our clients, and social and biological events seem to either support or challenge their lives, we as professional helpers serve to help create that mountain ground.

It takes a strong back to listen, become a part of the story, be expected by the client to help (yet be uncertain just how to do so), and to sincerely proceed even in the midst of not knowing—and allow your open, soft heart to work in tandem with your strong back. The strong back provides for stillness in the face of client winds that violently shake branches but do not disturb roots. The strong back is about practitioner patience, willingness to be uncertain, willingness to accept pain for what it is and not reflexively react so as to either "fix" the client or appease your own professional ego. When you *do* engage in action, the practitioner with a strong back incorporates calmness and balance. Panic, anger, reactivity do not govern your responses. The helper with a strong back is grounded enough that she or he does not flap around to suit the treatment fad of the day, or seek to please or impress clients or prestigious professionals so as to receive undeserved credit or pursue personal opportunities.

A still, settled mind characterizes the helping practitioner with a strong back, and this stillness exists even as the practitioner shifts perspectives or ways of being. The practitioner moves from spontaneity to deliberate, planned interventions; goes the extra mile, then pulls back to honor boundaries; bridges the treatment dialectic (to be discussed later) between radical acceptance and validation on the one hand and client change on the other, while she maintains a solidity and stability that makes her appear as if—as Zen teacher Reb Anderson says—"she is not moving even while she is moving."

Not moving in the midst of pain and an implicit client demand for relief or for solutions is about remaining still and letting the present expand as the client tells her story. This all may sound rhetorical—and often times throughout the book words and concepts will be poor substitutes for firsthand experience in capturing phenomena—so let us see how the strong back operates with a simple example. A distressed and concerned mother told me how her 14-year-old son had become increasingly difficult to discipline. He went on the run for 1 month to show his mother that there was no way he was going to move to a town 4 hours away and live with her and the boy's stepfather (of 4 years). He instead wanted to stay in town with his already established buddies and await the release of his father from prison. The mother told me that James' plan involved him and his father—who was convicted of selling marijuana—eventually establishing a household once his father left prison. As the mother discussed her son's plans and historical familial events, she was a flood of thoughts and feelings: *I am a failure as a mother for choosing to move with my husband and leave my son with his father* [though she did visit her ex-husband in jail to evaluate what kind of home he could possibly provide for her son]; *I should be able to just make him move—I am too soft for letting him make this decision; moving back and forth between these two homes is not good for my son—it is not what I ever wanted or imagined for him; I should have done a better job mediating between my son and his stepfather for the years they were together and James' stepfather unsuccessfully attempted to be a father figure; I have spoiled my son and now he is running the show and manipulating me; I don't know how things are going to turn out.*

In this storm of grief, resentment, doubt, confusion, guilt, and despair, there was an impotent social worker sitting across from this mother experiencing some of these emotions with her. I periodically tuned into my breath as I listened, sat up straight, and brought myself back to the sacred activity of listening. At times, I needed to check my inclination to dart about like a mouse crossing a busy kitchen, and I noticed my fleeting wishes to say something impressive or propose a solution. After all, this woman was suffering; through my inactivity I asked myself: *Am I appearing stupid to her?* Then I noticed that this was an arising thought. Noticing that this was nothing more than an arising thought meant that I did not have to become engrossed in the thought or feel compelled to react to the unpleasantness that the thought could have brought had I indulged it more completely. This was a powerful example of how mindfulness vis-à-vis my own process allowed me to stay present for the mother's story and pain rather than to shift to a reactive fight-or-flight response that would have rendered me ineffective. After watching this thought related to my own insecurities and, perhaps, discomfort from being in the midst of pain and emotional turmoil, a slight awareness of breath and posture brought me back to a place and time that I have learned to trust—the here and now.

## Trusting the Here and Now

In the here and now, or the present moment, profound and helpful questions, comments, ideas, and insights occur. As the present moment expands—as a result of the practitioner's reduced internal chatter and focus on maintaining a strong back—creativity, connection, curiosity, and helpfulness emerge. Martin Luther King believed that if he trusted the moment, God would speak through him. He learned that lesson during Montgomery's burgeoning bus boycott. Even in the midst of violent acts and threats committed against him and his family, as well as self-doubts concerning the best way to galvanize the movement, Dr. King believed that as he created peace within his own mind, he could count on the moment to provide him with what was needed. He opened his heart to the larger force that he called "God" and what Zen practitioners may call big mind, the Pure Land, Buddha, God, nirvana, emptiness, or the great unknown.

*What could I say to keep them courageous and prepared for positive action and yet devoid of hate and resentment?* King contemplated this question as a *koan*—a Zen riddle designed to deepen wisdom—with hardly any time to prepare one of his most important speeches. At the end of the speech, Dr. King realized he had successfully woven together the telling of the African American story in the South—a story of suffering and courage, with a forceful, compelling, moral argument insisting on the end of suffering—"there comes a time when people get tired of being trampled over by the iron feet of oppression . . . when people get tired of being pushed out of the glittering sunlight of life's July, and left standing amid the piercing chill of an alpine November" (Carson, 1998, p. 60).

King reflected on his speech that night in Montgomery:

> As I sat listening to the continued applause I realized that this speech had evoked more response than any speech or sermon I had ever delivered. I came to see for the first time what the older preachers meant when they said, open your mouth and God will speak for you. (Carson, 1998, p. 61)

The Zen story about dynamics with clients is a variation of Dr. King's account. Trust that if you bring yourself with a strong back to the present moment, you will tap into the universe's reservoir of wisdom and skillful means. Just like Dr. King let God speak for him, when you, the practitioner, are genuine, grounded, calm, and connected to the other, skillful questions, statements, actions, nonverbal communication, and heartfelt interventions arise. To an extent—in Zen—it is not the helping practitioner who separately and independently decides how to act. Sure it seems that way, but helping professional actions emerge from the entire, universal constellation of actions and factors related to the practitioner's own life, historical and immediate lessons, learned theories and perspectives, the client's presence, words, emotions, and characteristics, and agency settings, and so on. The practitioner is a conduit for these universal forces in a similar manner that Dr. King was a conduit for God on that night in Montgomery. We may even say that clinical practice or any kind of helping practice for that matter is about getting out of our own way and dropping the self.

Let us get back to James' mother whom we refer to as Ms. Smith. In the midst of Ms. Smith's self-denigrating comments about how she had lost control of her son, there were many directions that I could have pursued. I could have asked Ms. Smith how she came to embrace these beliefs about herself and then either had her examine the beliefs' validity or directly challenge the beliefs myself. I could have explored the areas of her relationship with her son and crafted solution-focused language relying on positive past successes and asked her what it would look like if her level of discipline effectiveness moved from a 3 out of 10 to a 5 or 6 out of 10. Then I could have followed up with questions about what it would take to make this improvement happen and set contracted-on tasks that related to these spelled-out discipline improvements.

Instead, I allowed Ms. Smith to grieve about her difficulties with her son. I joined with her regarding the difficulties that she had experienced being in the middle of her son and her second husband as well as her son and her first husband: I admired her courage for trying to do the best for her son and for telling her story even in the midst of her own self-judgments about her family's life. I told her that I have seen youth rise to the occasion even as they go back and forth between two different households, as I have seen youth crumble even while their household looks "normal" to the outside world. "Your sincerity, honesty, love, and willingness to stay committed during the hard times is the best you can do right now, and although it is hard to accept, you ultimately have no control of the outcome," was more or less what I said. I summarized my understanding of her son's positive qualities, including his caring phone contacts with her that occurred even during the time that he had run away. I added, "and that *story* you have about what an inadequate mom you are because you have not done the right things or have not correctly disciplined your son—JUST DROP IT!"

"Thank you," she said, as her load appeared to lighten. She left my office seeming calm and settled about her son's initiating contact with me. I gave her some tips on not selling me as a therapist—so that her son could make a ruling on me that was not clouded by her perceptions—and we set up an appointment time that would have the greatest likelihood for success, deciding that a weekend would be best (despite my desire not to work on weekends).

## Uncertainty of Interventions

To what degree was my decision to create space allowing Ms. Smith to grieve part of my orientation regarding the importance of becoming aware of the deep truth about one's present experience? Joan Halifax, in fact, says things like: "Without going into the darkness, we project it into the landscape" (see Halifax, 1993). Although I like to think of myself as being open, flexible, and spontaneous, I do carry with me the paradigm that "the truth will set you free" and that truth in our clients' situations often involves mucking around in the mud of their lives. Does my mandate for her to drop her self-deprecating story contradict her being able to experience her grief? How much did these words come from my clever assessment of what would be the most helpful to Ms. Smith and her child? And how much did they emerge from my own experience of permissively raising special needs children and my own process of slowly letting a story line go that I told Ms. Smith she needed to immediately drop? Do my personal experiences provide powerful insight opportunities or counter-transference land mines or both? Was my decision to point out the strengths of her son part of my strengths orientation as a social worker, or part of what I think was especially important in this particular instance and/or what I, myself, wish to hear as a parent?

It is clear that no matter what reductionist proponents say about evidence-based practice, there are countless nuances related to this work and no one way to proceed. The client's story, circumstances, and presentation dynamically interact with the practitioner's story, circumstances, mood, strong back, and open heart moment to moment. Not only are we uncertain about the eventual outcomes, if we are really honest, we are not even certain about the process. Our strong back creates the walls of the container where the client feels that she or he can explore thoughts, feelings, circumstances, hardships, triumphs, and stories. Our strong back keeps us rooted and helpful; if it were not for this strength, clients and practitioners would engage in mutual spinning, flapping, flailing, obsessing, running, hiding, freezing, or perseverating. Our strong back provides the foundation for us to enter the unknown and uncertain—the place where suffering exists and the ways out are not yet illumined. With our strong back, we are prepared to love our clients even in the midst of darkness; we maintain the stance that the best place to be is right here, even though there is so little we can count on.

## SOFT FRONT

As mentioned, the strong back is the ground for the soft front, or open heart. The soft front refers to the practitioner's open-hearted disposition toward the client as well as for him or herself. Our soft front allows us to be truly touched by our clients' lives. We begin to actually experience our clients' pain, because as we sit—open-hearted—with our clients, we deeply realize that their pain is ultimately the world's pain; we do not shy away from this connection. Soft-heartedness in the midst of pain defies our frequent response to pain that Stephen Levine describes as sending hatred or aversion rather than mercy or compassion to our wounded heart.

Cultivating an open heart requires that we be patient and still. We maintain curiosity and we hesitate before intellectualizing and categorizing. In a manner that is difficult to explain, being open-hearted requires us to feel spacious and to go to the room in the house that does not have the chattering mind. I will provide a self-care example that, although not directly a social service or therapy situation, is illustrative.

### Open Heart and Mindfulness

During the time leading up to my writing today, I was feeling pretty depressed. It was at the end of a day and I was tired. I scanned the house and saw the messy piles of clothes and grungy bathroom floors. I began perseverating about my children, making mental notes of their various difficulties and challenges, then I started weaving a story about how difficult our family life is. The depression seemed to generate thoughts and stories that made the depression ever more solid and all-encompassing. I started perseverating about all the things that I did not accomplish today, and judged myself as being too lazy and emotionally paralyzed to get back to writing. I started thinking about trips that I could perhaps take because, after all, I surely deserved one. As my mind was building a monument to depression, I spread out on my unmade bed and stared at the patterns on the ceiling. One thought did, however, provide a key to recovery. I did not have to attach myself to this cycle of thinking; the antidote was to let it all be spacious. Breathing deeply and tuning into my breath brought me to a state of spaciousness that was not conducive for preserving and contributing to the monument of depression that had been constructed. Personal feeling states and thoughts tightly woven and so imposing that it felt like all of life was these oppressive feelings and thoughts began to dissolve into the spaciousness of breath. Clarity emerged and I was able to see the depression and the supporting or generating thoughts for what they were—feeling states and impermanent thoughts. I began to feel not so sorry for myself and to think of myself in less pathetic terms. The way I had been feeling—which had seemed so solid, global, and formidable—was loosening its grip. The steady stream of thoughts that accompanied my mood slowed down; I could see the thoughts for what they were—mental formations—and I began to let them go. My heart opened up to myself, my family, and to the beautiful photo of Martin Luther King on the cover of his autobiography. I lovingly stepped away from the laptop computer and made my son a cheese sandwich and felt transformed.

The open heart trusts the present moment as well. It tunes into love for self and other and recognizes the divinity or karma that has brought you and this client together. The slow, mindful breath breathes life into the open or soft heart. The heart stays soft as the chatter related to whom the client is, what your responses need to be, what you may be feeling, and how you may be performing remains a quiet whisper. As the chatter becomes ever more quiet, you develop a deep nonintellectualized sense that the essence of the other involving breath, energy, emotions, involuntary processes, and life force are completely shared with you. You realize that the clients sitting across from you wear behaviors, stories, problems, characteristics as adornments or—as James Baraz says, "magical displays," that can distract you into thinking that these observances are the actual human beings themselves. These magical displays and practitioner stories or assessments about the displays can remove you from the essence of the other that involves her or his light, love, or divinity.

The thinking, scheming mind builds all kinds of monuments. In this example, my mind built a monument to depression; what the mind typically builds in helping professionals are monuments to certainty, so-called evidenced-based knowledge, or brilliant interventions. As our thoughts are spinning away, we experience our clients as others whom we do something to. Our hearts begin to close to their actual experience or nature of their struggles and to who they in fact are. We may even adopt a hard and constricted front as our shared hurts are covered by our own frustrations and anger toward our clients for not being who we wish they would be. We resort to familiar labels, such as "manipulative" or "inappropriate," that reflect our frustrations with our clients for their not doing the things we think are best for them or for not upholding the rules or protocols.

We see them as separate from us and do not realize that, save for some good fortune, our stories could be identical. We also fail to see that on a certain level we and our clients are walking together. Our lives are ultimately linked and the most naked proof of this is that we are in the same room, sitting over the same story, and we both want the client's happiness.

## CONTEMPLATION EXERCISE

Slow down your pace of reading this book and begin to tune into your slow, calm breath.

Soften your heart to the reality of your interdependence with clients. Soften your heart to the universal nature of pain, how archetypal it is, and how, therefore, no one owns it. The river of pain that is passing through your client now is the same river that passes through you, though yours has different twists and turns and, perhaps, different levels of depth or strength of current. Let yourself feel—in your heart—the ultimate purpose of your work and your ultimate connection to "the other." As you sit down with a client or as you read this book, consistently ask yourself, "What brings me here?" As you imagine yourself taking your seat in the presence of your client, let your breath connect you with your client. The air you breathe is not yours, there is no "you" or individual "I" who is breathing. Our nondivisibility is evident when we deeply tune into our surroundings.

### Barriers to Strong Back/Soft Front Work:
### Evidence-Based Practice

You have not been encouraged to practice with a soft heart. You have probably been taught that, in fact, soft-heartedness is equivalent to nonprofessionalism and poor boundaries. Some may question whether soft-heartedness runs counter to empowering clients, and we discuss the empowerment issue in Chapter 3 on radical acceptance. Counseling, psychology, social work, and other helping professions are not going to rush to embrace soft-heartedness. The whole idea sounds too wimpy, looks too intellectually unimpressive, and seems too unscientific compared to professions, particularly medicine, that do not have nearly the same credibility challenges.

The newest incarnation of various helping professions' never-ending quest for credibility has taken the form of framing all kinds of work as "evidence-based practice." Helping professions increasingly adopt the pretence that it is not so much an issue of whether we are engaging in open-hearted work. What is most important is that we work from a place of knowing. We are to pretend that helping practice is not about negotiating our way through uncertainty or the unknown but is about shrinking the unknown and working within realms of greater and greater degrees of certainty. We are supposed to be less about strong backs and soft fronts in our journeys with clients and more about accurate client profiling and prescribed interventions.

In an article appearing in *Social Work*, McNeill (2006) argued against social constructivism, stating that:

> the social world is still knowable even if in incomplete ways. . . . Ultimately, this world may be interpreted uniquely by each individual, but it is knowable in the sense that there may be more or less evidence about it and *agreement on a collective level*. (p. 149, italics mine)

In other words, when there was strong agreement within professional circles that homosexuality was pathological, was that *non*relativistic knowledge? Suppose there had been research documenting higher sexual confusion rates, more promiscuous behavior, and higher rates of suicide for gays and lesbians. Would these studies have contributed to the *knowledge* of homosexual client pathology?

There are many reasons why a positivist orientation is out of step with the realities of our work. Although I present some of the limitations of evidence-based work, not all diagnostic schemes and so-called expert knowledge are useless. My own experience as a practitioner and parent has taught me about the possibilities of a traditional clinical response to various situations. It is the worshipping of and attachment to medical or so-called evidence-based models and the relative ignorance of broader paradigms that is problematic for the helping professions as well as for the clients whom these professionals serve.

On the most general level, the language of evidence-based practice symbolizes the kind of invisibility that clients are accustomed to—especially the low-income and disenfranchised clients community-based practitioners often serve. Helping professional discourse now devalues client-centered approaches in lieu of evidence-based rhetoric. Rarely does the evidence have to do with client satisfaction but with so-called objective indicators of behaviors or feeling states. We are to pitch our interactions with clients to meet targets or outcomes rather than to address and deal with clients who are in pain and who often are not sure if they want to trust us or even be in the same room with us. The following example illustrates this:

> As I met with James, I decided to ask him to leave the office with me to get a soda. I later asked him to write for me about the pros and cons of smoking marijuana and he happily agreed, vowing to start writing an essay that evening.

Will walking outside and buying James a soda more likely lead to positive outcomes? Should I be more confrontive in the third session about James' marijuana use rather than have him write an essay, the process of which utilizes a stated skill and provides me an opportunity to acknowledge his strengths as a writer? Am I spending too much time talking to James about sports? He has talked about being part American Indian: should I refer him to a sweat lodge ceremony? Am I swearing too much or should I follow a model regarding language that is more consistent with his school environment? I wanted to let James have some control over the process, and I asked him whether he wanted to see me each week or every other week. Should I have asked him this question or should I have been the one to establish a more parental boundary and define the nature of our interaction more definitively? Should I interpret it as a step toward success when he stated that he wanted to come every week or should I consider that until he stops smoking marijuana we can not think in terms of successes?

When we are tuned into the nature of this work, we understand that these kinds of unanswerable questions form its ground. How we negotiate, move through, embrace, and thrive in uncertainty determines our moment-to-moment as well as our long-term successes. At the same time, it is important to be aware of how our "agreements" about what constitutes knowledge or best practices (McNeill, 2006) are fluid and forever changing, are based on incomplete and sometimes contrived studies and measures, and may have little or nothing to do with the client sitting across from you or for that matter what can possibly be practiced within the confines of your service setting.

The increasing objectification and distillation of our clients' lives into outcome measures parallels the developments in education where "No Child Left Behind" is actually about "No Test Score Left Behind." The cultural underpinnings that rule the day concerning public education and human service are strikingly similar and seem to include: (a) conservative policymaker distrust of helping or teaching professionals, (b) infusion of economic-oriented philosophy and terminology concerning the purpose of the endeavor, (c) formation of a segment of university researchers who elevate numbers-driven service provision or kindergarten through 12 education as virtuous and responsible while labeling practitioners and educators at the direct service level as backward and unscientific, and (d) objectification of the kindergarten through 12 children or service recipients.

"The children are invisible," one experienced, well-respected educator exclaimed in the middle of a workshop I gave at an elementary school. The school process is organized to yield a better product—that is, higher test scores—while the curriculum, teacher creativity, and discussion related to child *education*, enrichment, and motivation has been deadened and rendered irrelevant. In the end, the more affluent will receive either private school educations or enrichment experiences that eschew or at the very least supplement the evidenced-based, test score curriculum that is reducing education to standardized curriculum packages, time on task mandates, and deletion of enrichments. The more affluent will similarly find their way to mental health practitioners who reject one-size-fits-all evidence-based models, who embrace clients for their uniqueness, and who enter into relationships with clients with a strong intention of deeply listening to each person's voice within a sacred space of not knowing.

## PARTNERSHIPS WITH CLIENTS/NOT WITH PRACTICE MODELS

> There are moments when rules
> are meant to be broken; when
> bursting out of context is the
> sole way to see with new eyes.
> There are fences built only to
> be torn down. The slats look
> solid, but no one drove the nails
> in tight. There are barricades
> around the heart asking to be
> breached. Sooner or later
> we all run out of excuses for
> staying small and safe.
> —Danna Faulds

This book emphasizes a process rooted in Zen thought that provides direction for us to be effectively present for our clients. Ultimately, our strong back and soft front as well as our radical acceptance, mindfulness, and open-heartedness help us effectively engage in partnerships with clients. I made the argument that an over-emphasis on evidence-based practice obscures the role of the *practitioner* as well as the importance of our internal gifts and process. Duncan, Miller, and Sparks (2004) argue from the other end, that evidence-based practice

> totally excludes the *client* from consideration. Its promoters equate the client with the problem and describe the treatment as if it is isolated from the most powerful factors that contribute to change—the client's resources, perceptions, and participation. (pp. 38–39, italics mine)

These authors suggest that in the therapeutic context, the client-practitioner *relationship* is the most powerful predictor of positive outcomes. Citing Asay and Lambert (1999), they state that client perceptions of the client-worker relationship accounts for 30% of the successful outcome. They present a meta-analysis study (Wampold, 2001) that suggests that 54% of the *variance* in client outcomes is attributable to the practitioner-client relationship. Other client-related factors involving hope, expectancy, and placebo effects and "extra-therapeutic" components including social support and ecological circumstances all together account for 55% of change. In a number of studies, the choice of the therapeutic model accounted for no more than 15% of the change in therapy.

The client-specific factors—persistence, openness, and optimism may be influenced through involvement in a positive helping relationship. For example, the degree to which the helper is seen as credible enhances the client factors. The therapy relationship factors themselves are identified as the practitioner's respect, empathic understanding, attentive listening, and friendliness.

Duncan et al. (2004) propose that practitioners view our clients as "heroic." We are not to minimize client pain or struggle but we listen for resilience and courage. Similar to a solution-focused stance, they suggest that we learn about client successes in an arena that appears problem-embedded. We ask clients to tell us about exceptions—"those past experiences . . . when the problem might reasonably have been expected to occur but somehow did not" (DeJong & Berg, 2002, p. 104). "What was happening at those times (during the exceptions)? What do you think you were doing to help that along?" (Duncan et al., 2004, p. 57).

We notice change and constantly applaud it. We inquire about and make special notice of gains that clients make session-to-session, and we explore changes that even occurred from the time the client made the appointment to the time she or he came to the first session (Duncan et al., 2004).

We enthusiastically connect with clients and open ourselves to their voice and their feedback. *We emphasize effectiveness over competence.* Effective relationships include actively learning from the client about his or her nuanced life and about what is or is not working in the relationship with the practitioner. In this regard, we seek what Duncan et al. (2004) refer to as "practice-based evidence" during our time with clients so that we can be accountable and responsive. We keep our eyes on the prize—actually helping the client, rather than dedicating our efforts toward practice competence—which is de-contextualized and not nearly as helpful.

Duncan et al. (2004) state:

> We must set aside the intellectual appeal of theoretical models, the promises of flashy techniques, the charisma of masters, and the marketing acumen of snake oil peddlers. The research indicates that therapy works if clients experience the relationship positively and are active participants. (pp. 36–37)

I believe that *The Zen of Helping* complements the orientation found in *The Heroic Client* even though Duncan et al. (2004) eschew a helping profession emphasis on process (and by process, they refer to the relative importance placed on technique or treatment theory over addressing case-specific client outcomes). The *Heroic Client* calls for practitioners to *partner with clients*, and develop a *relational bond*—which directly or indirectly includes the practitioner's acceptance, validation, flexibility, responsiveness, self-disclosure, creativity, alertness, friendship, collaboration, and nondefensiveness in the face of client-expressed dissatisfaction. Additionally, because their notions of practice conflict with the helping professions' evidence-based culture, they implicitly call for practitioners to be willing to go against the grain and, to some extent, be heroic themselves. *The Zen of Helping* directly addresses the ways in which practitioners contribute to creating the positive helping relationships called for in the *Heroic Client*.

Duncan et al. (2004) encourage us to move our attention from the abstract and sometimes nonapplicable world of theoretical models to the nuanced aspirations, needs, and possibilities of clients. They inspire us to look at the real person who is sitting across from us—our client. Our strong back and soft front—as well as the other spiritual principles within these pages—moves us to look at and embody the other real person in the room—yourself. *Our relational work demands an effective focus on both parts of the equation—client and practitioner—and I maintain that we have severely neglected the practitioner side of the coin.*

The following questions are important for practitioners to consider in order to serve the "Heroic Client" within an effective partnership:

- How do we stay centered, responsive, accepting, and open-hearted when clients provide feedback that we are not doing a good job?
- How do we keep our hearts open and listen for strengths and resilience when the client has already been defined as pathological or has actively rebelled against us or acted out in some manner?
- How do we maintain our client-practitioner partnership when judgments—as they always do—arise within us?
- Given that the client is attuned to our level of caring, how do we "bring it" when our energy is low?
- How do we negotiate boundaries while the client wishes to experience qualities of friendship?
- How do we bear witness and hold our ground in the face of client trauma? How do we know whether our focus on outcomes is a client-centered response or practitioner flight from client pain?
- When does tuning into the "client's theory of change" just another practitioner agenda that possibly disconnects us from the client's desire to simply be heard or accepted for who she is?
- How do we transcend the duality of illness versus resilience/strength and: (a) see that these apparent polarities may be two sides of the coin—that is, not mutually exclusive, and (b) embrace that sometimes a label or diagnosis creates possibilities for client relief or benefit.
- How do we connect with our clients when we are afraid?
- How do we balance open-heartedness with strong back confrontation and limit-setting?

## MANDATED CLIENTS

There are particular dynamics more often found with mandated clients that also deserve mentioning. In these cases, the client's theory of change may be: "The less you (the practitioner) find out about me the safer I will be." Another client theory of change may be: "The more I can act like this program is meaningful to me, the sooner I can graduate and start using drugs again." With these kinds of perspectives, the feedback we receive about our helping efforts may be along the lines of: "Get out of my @#%! business. . . . I don't want your bag of tricks." Or we may receive responses that are more polite but fundamentally express a deep suspicion, irritation, and reluctance to engage in the helping process.

These situations are complicated with the reality that our "client" may also be the state in the form of Child Protective Services, a probation department, a public school, or drug treatment diversion program. Sometimes we are working with a parent who wishes to get her children returned to her; however, we are ultimately responsible for the safety of the children so our treatment involves our "assessment" of the parent's readiness for parenting. We work with great patience and compassion for ourselves and our clients in these circumstances. The environment inevitably produces conflicts for us to navigate. We would like to be client-centered and maintain a high level of confidentiality; yet we consistently interject our strong back so that the client maintains accountability. Compromised confidentiality defines the service context right from the beginning, and the client may understandably not trust the process. In a context that is characterized by suspicion and fear, we stay mindful of not becoming suspicious and fearful ourselves and not establishing a service culture of us versus them.

We realize how much uncertainty and ambiguity defines our moment-to-moment interactions in these settings. Even following a paradigm such as "client-directed, outcome-informed therapy" (Duncan et al., 2004) does not diminish the reality that not-knowing characterizes our work. We learn to embrace not-knowing and we move ahead with a soft front and strong back.

Cultivating and maintaining a strong back and soft or open front is enormously challenging. We all have experienced conditioning that leads us to move and react in the face of difficulty (fight-or-flight) and to send fear or anger to our wounded heart rather than sit with a client's (as well as our own) pain as it is. Additionally, as we have discussed, this society often prefers to construct illusory certainty rather than maintain a strong back in the midst of not knowing. In fact, one may say that decision making by the leaders in this country is unfortunately characterized by a weak back and hard front.

The rest of the book will be a call for you to open your heart, be authentic, and, with clarity, enter the present moment with your clients. As we explore various topics related to the *Zen of Helping*, you will see that the book suggests a journey that demands effort, as well as a willingness to be vulnerable and to not know. I have already seen how students and practitioners benefit from seriously reflecting on this book's concepts and experimenting with integrating them into their work. Consider the possibility that your engagement with this material is transformative and that applying sincere effort impacts the presence and effectiveness that you will have with your clients. Here are some opportunities for further engagement:

- When you engage in a classroom discussion or small group exercise, notice what it means to sit with a strong back and soft front. Even though it may feel awkward at first, sit up straight in your chair and open your chest so that you embody a strong back and soft front.
- Reflect on your tendencies or comfort level with either a strong back or a soft front. Reflect on and/or discuss the ways in which a strong back and soft front are mutually reinforcing.
- Maintain awareness of your strong back and soft front with clients, groups, and during staff or community meetings. How does the notion of strong back and soft front prepare you to deal with the various challenges related to relationship-building, finding out information (assessment), and intervention?
- Reflect on the degree to which you feel liberated and/or fearful about how much we do not know while we are engaged in practice.
- How much are you able to relax with not knowing? Take note of times in helping relationships and in your social or family life where moments arise and no clear direction is evident.

Part of our strong back involves tuning into our intentions, then making a decision to bring our focused energy to learn, take risks, and grow. We "burst out of context" as suggested in the poem on page 21—that often involves our passivity and our inclination to skate along the surface—and bring ourselves into this present moment acting as if nothing else in the world is as important. And nothing else is! We approach the contemplations and exercises suggested as well as the material throughout the book with the conscious intention to meet our life. This strong back conviction provides the container for our flourishing soft front. As we open our hearts to this journey, it will be increasingly clear that freedom—for ourselves and our clients—represents the essence of the discussions and opportunities found throughout the book. Why not begin now?

# Chapter Three

# RADICAL ACCEPTANCE OF CLIENTS, CONTEXT, AND SELF

*Beyond Carl Rogers' Positive Regard*

Beautiful ground for our work occurs when we experience complete, unconditional acceptance for our clients. Professionals are often quick to say that they accept their clients, but the kind of acceptance spoken about here is quite profound and perhaps different than what you have experienced or heard about before. Radical acceptance is not only about being non-judgmental; its nature refers to the practitioner's felt experience and to the practitioner's intent to establish a field of unconditional love for the client. Radical acceptance of clients requires more than flipping a radical acceptance switch in your mind. Sustained effort and mindfulness are required to radically accept clients. Radical acceptance of our clients and our clients' circumstances represents the soft front that feeds and bolsters the strong back required for navigating uncertain waters. This chapter discusses the nature of radical acceptance as well as its benefits. Then we examine some practice applications.

On the most basic level, radical acceptance involves a deep appreciation for the other, which is experienced cognitively, emotionally, and spiritually. Appreciation takes the form of truly enjoying the presence of the other person and sensing, experiencing, and believing that life is better because of the existence of that individual. These elements are similar to the perspective of Carl Rogers (1961) who advanced the notion of unconditional positive regard.

The orientation presented here transcends Rogers in that: (a) radical acceptance is a moment-to-moment experience involving *the practitioner's own process and arising thoughts and emotions* as well as acceptance of the client; (b) there is a body experience rooted in the breath that creates a field of acceptance in addition to the mental, contemplative processes that Rogers emphasized; and (c) radical acceptance is spiritually rooted.

Although a client may be difficult to be with and some may be tempted to label this individual as uncooperative, lazy, manipulative, or, worse, borderline or antisocial, I see this person as a divine being who has qualities that I, myself, could have manifested had I had the same kinds of experiences, bad luck, traumas, biology, and so on. What a gift that I have an opportunity to be with this beautiful being who, for whatever reason, was handed a different pair of shoes than me and to some degree either chose or was pushed to walk down a difficult path. Thich Nhat Hanh (1999) expresses this sentiment most poignantly in a poem entitled "Call Me by My True Names." We are the victims of the most heinous crimes and we are the perpetrators. We all possess the nature and capacity to behave violently and cruelly as well as the capacity to love and live a life of compassion and service. Because in our lives seeds of either joy and compassion or ignorance and greed were more or less watered, we developed inclinations to think, act, and feel in one way or another.

Unfortunately, we often ignore—or are ignorant of—how our nature and our inherent capacities are affected by causes and conditions (karma). We ignore how this being who is called "I" relies on the same air, water, space, and substances as the one we think of as "other," and we ignore that, in fact, we do not independently will ourselves into existence nor can we independently prevent the demise of our particular body. Ignoring or being ignorant of how we are not separate, independent selves affects our sense of the other in the midst of a client-professional relationship. If you buy into the view that you, as a practitioner, and the client are completely independent, separate selves, then you are vulnerable to having disdain for the client for not measuring up to your standards. You may not appreciate how *your* pain is actually a window into the *client's* pain and that the universal and archetypal nature of pain and suffering actually means that it does not belong per se to *any particular* being. The universal river of pain and suffering is flowing through the space that you and the client occupy, and pain and suffering flow through the universe as do other feeling states, thought configurations, and behavioral patterns. As client and practitioner beings, your bodies, Buddhist psychologist Jack Kornfield says, are renting these universal forces, including the force called life.

## THE RELATIVE AND THE ABSOLUTE

This kind of orientation is typically puzzling and runs counter to our conditioning, particularly in Western society where notions of me and freedom of the individual are sacred. Even the professions of social work and counseling bestow particular virtue on *individuating* youth, *self-determined* clients, and *independent* living for people with disabilities. A Zen Buddhist would say that a perspective that recognizes the importance of the individual and stresses how one person is the practitioner with one name and the other is the client with another name incorporates a *relative* or *conventional* view of existence. This view is helpful for us because all beings need to negotiate issues related to survival and health and thus we rely on a story about life that emphasizes reality as it appears on face value. This face value story is typically embraced in Western thought as *the only story*. One individual tries to make sense of the world on a unique path with or without the help of family or friends or a guide. A practitioner working within this paradigm becomes more focused on maintaining healthy I-and-thou boundaries rather than appreciating mutual interdependence. The Judeo-Christian spiritual perspective often is in accord with this I-and-thou view: God is seen as residing outside the individual and it is the individual's task in life to "get right with God" so as to reap the rewards that the separate entity—God—will bestow on him or her.

The other story about the nature of existence emphasizes the fundamental, nonseparate nature of existence. As the Zen helping practitioner enters the room with a client, she senses how all beings are universally sacred creatures and/or embodiments of God, spirit, the great unknown or "Big Mind." People in the East, for example, may bow to one another to acknowledge the presence of the divine in each. In the radical acceptance tradition, one may figuratively bow to the client to affirm the blessing that this individual client is exactly who she or he is. Additionally, the practitioner accepts her own limitations, strengths, areas of confusion, and feelings, and while with the client fully embraces the one thing that Zen teacher Joko Beck says you can count on—that "life is being as it is." We can refer to the elements of this story of interdependence and radical acceptance as a description of *absolute reality*.

How do we rectify our treasured Western notions of self and the self's relation to mental health with the Zen Buddhist orientation that belief in a separate self is a foundation of ignorance and world suffering? Nondualistic thought, a cornerstone of Eastern thinking, is our way out of this conundrum. We discuss the issue of dialectics in a later chapter, but for now let us say that *the task is to hold both realities—the relative and the absolute—as two sides of the same coin.* Each side is essential to the coin and one view does not supersede the other. Typically in Western discourse, complex issues are depicted as dualities: strengths perspective versus medical model, positivism versus social constructionism, color-blind versus cultural competence, and so on. Here, just as we see later, both so-called opposite views are simultaneously held. As Thich Nhat Hanh discusses, we see the individual chocolate chip cookies and know that they appear separate and that, with their chocolate chip minds, they compare themselves to one another, and we also know that each cookie was made from the same batter; thus, their view regarding their independent separateness is an illusion.

How do we experience the cookies in a nondualistic way? We see the cookies' unique qualities and how some are eaten one at a time while some are put away in the cookie jar. We count as we eat each one and notice that some are smaller or larger, more or less burned and perhaps, as a result, more or less appetizing. We see our hands touch the cookies and notice the clear separation or boundary between hand and cookie. This is the relative or conventional view. At the same time, we look deeply into each cookie's existence, and we understand that their origin lies in the batter bowl before they were dropped one spoonful at a time on to the cookie sheet. As we look deeper, we are intimately aware that these things called cookies are made up of various components—flour, butter, chips, baking powder, and so on, as well as the human effort that went into making the cookies as well as the oven. The flour comes from wheat that relies on water to grow. Human beings rely on water as do the cookies and this water comes from clouds and rivers and so on. This is the absolute view of reality. Being nondualistic means that we do not argue about which way is more right or accurate—the absolute or the relative. (In advanced Zen, we become aware that ultimately these views themselves are mere stories about existence and not existence itself.) We cling to neither story, but embrace the stories as they are, and in a way act as if they are simultaneously true.

Thus, through a relative lens, we understand that there is a client and a practitioner, that the notion of healthy boundaries (which we discuss later) is important and helpful, and that each one's narrative is unique and needs to be heard and validated as if it were unique. At the same time, through an absolute lens, we approach our clients attuned to the sacred and boundless space of life where, as Thich Nhat Hanh says, *the sun is our heart.* The overall field of radical acceptance is inclusive enough that both relative and absolute perspectives are embraced. The coin cannot exist without each of the sides, and the existence of one of the sides is completely interdependent on the existence of the other.

This sense of interdependence permeates the practitioner-client relationship. Not only are the client's life and my life interdependent by virtue of our mutual paths as human beings, but on a basic level, I rely on the client's presence to have an occupation and a sense of meaningful contribution. In this field of interdependence or the absolute, I am especially aware of artificial barriers such as professional and client, the mentally healthy and the mentally unhealthy, the expert and the client or student. In this boundless place, I love this client as I love the universe. I encounter peace regarding what is, and I experience an open heart and the health that derives from being unattached to outcomes. Radical acceptance then becomes an openhearted spiritual, emotional, and intellectual journey with a client that simultaneously embraces the relative world of boundaries, goals, or outcomes, and at times, diagnostic labels. In a state of radical acceptance, one accepts the difficulties and imperfectly resolved contradictions that arise when absolute and relative views bump into each other.

## RADICAL ACCEPTANCE AND YOU

Radical acceptance ultimately provides the container for your relationship with your clients as well as with yourself. Instead of judgments related to your personal superiority, a personal agenda to make the client be other than he or she is, or personal despair, disgust, or frustration regarding the client's behavior infiltrating your being, radical acceptance allows you to serenely engage with a soft front and with a wide appreciation of your common human condition. Radical acceptance provides the ground to inquire with curiosity and learn from your clients; to be inspired by your client's story; and to feel compassionate, patient, and forgiving. When clients experience your radical acceptance of them, they become disposed to explore their inner and outer lives with you. They move through this healing space with you secure in the knowledge that you accept them exactly as they are.

Maintaining radical acceptance for clients (or for coworkers, for that matter) is especially challenging when they, themselves, are so nonaccepting of others. I often see parents scoff at their children's sincere expression of emotional turmoil and pain and seek to make their children's pain disappear through strategies of minimization, denial, accusation, and dismissal. It seems that parents become nonaccepting because they have been so burdened with their children's pain that they are driven to not let their children's pain penetrate them. Well-intentioned and loving parents will actually giggle and smirk when their children talk to them during family sessions about how difficult and desperate their lives are and how frustrated they are when their parents do not seem to listen. The practitioner's ability to be radically accepting is truly put to the test when parental nonacceptance and even hurtful behavior is unveiled right in your midst.

"Can we talk about that (facial) expression?" I asked as I observed a mother look away in apparent disgust as her depressed 13-year-old son talked about how he wished she would truly listen to his difficulties rather than exhorting him to take a walk outside. "Your son is talking about something that is painful in his life, and it seems that it is difficult for you to hear it," I said. In this moment, I felt loving toward this mom. Life is hard if this is the best she can do at this moment. She is either stuck in a pattern because her behavioral repertoire is limited or because she is not skillful and/or emotionally strong enough to effectively be present for her son's pain. There also may be a part of her that, because she loves her son so, deeply wishes that his pain could be resolved through unconscious strategies of denial or minimization.

In a space of radical acceptance, I talk with the mom about how important it is to listen to each other in the session. I am not there to judge, like in a court of law; I expect everyone's descriptions of given events to be different. The facts about what happened, however, are not nearly as important as listening for the essence of how different situations are experienced. I add that parents never want to see their child in pain. "We care about our kids and we want their pain to be gone, and it hurts us to witness their suffering. As a result, we sometimes try to offer simple solutions, tell our children to look on the bright side, or even push them away in an attempt to not have their pain add to our own. It is so hard and sometimes hurtful to just listen knowing that we may not have an answer for the child. This kind of listening, although challenging, is what your son needs from you."

This direct and fairly confrontational intervention emerged from the ground of radical acceptance for this mother. Although other practitioners had suggested that she was manipulative and narcissistic, I felt nothing but the highest regard for this beautiful being and her tangled story, her struggles to survive, her mistakes, shortcomings, and sincerity. She looked into my eyes warmly as the session concluded and thanked me. Her husband clearly experienced gratitude for her behavior change, which was visible throughout the session. The 13-year-old son said that she was doing a nice job of listening in the session, but he did not think it would carry over. At which point she told him, "You will see, it will be different."

Cultivating radical acceptance of your clients necessitates that you radically accept yourself. Your clients come to you for some relief from their struggles and pain. Even the involuntary ones come to you so they can escape the pain of losing their children to Child Protective Services or the pain of anticipated punishment for not complying. In the midst of *their* quest for a degree of liberation, you may be sitting with them constricted and bound up in your own issues: insecurities, irritations, doubts, ego-trips, frustrations, fantasies, or counter-transference reactions. You may be doing good, constructive work, but then suddenly find yourself in the middle of a session, spending time indulging yourself with beliefs about how smart you were for coming up with a particular intervention.

These thoughts and feelings do not contribute to—and may detract from—the task at hand. Within a field of radical acceptance, you, the practitioner, forgive yourself for distractions. This process allows you to move on from your own personal discourses and twisted emotions in order to stay present with your client.

Practitioner self-acceptance does not promote distractions. Instead, radical acceptance of the practitioner's self sets the ground for "letting go" of unproductive thoughts or feelings. For example, let us say I have an initial meeting with a client and after a short time I start to feel insecure about her rage and inadequate because my engagement with her does not seem to be reducing her agitation. As a result of my insecurity and self-judgment, I find myself inclined to search for mental health labels that can justify my futility more than tuning into her pain. In a field of radical self-acceptance, I observe my own process. I do not react to how the session has unfolded, I see my self-absorption for what it has been, I deeply smile to myself, and move on. My deep smile reflects love and forgiveness for my fallibilities. My deep smile reflects the mental, bodily, and spiritual recognition that this session unfolded just as it did—there is no going back and changing it. My deep smile is there for my client as well. Her anger . . . my insecurity . . . our uncertainty . . . our shared journey . . . our propensities to rush to judgment . . . and our mutual need for understanding are all in the room as we sit together. I become thoroughly grounded in the realization that tuning into this woman's pain and hearing her story is what she is here for, even though professional and scholarly discourses value the categorization of her complex life.

Radical acceptance of my own process has quieted what Buddhist psychologist Tara Brach (2003) describes as "the trance of unworthiness." Ironically, our skillfulness at identifying and accepting this trance ultimately strips it of its power. As I breathe calmly and see the manifestation of this trance for what it is—in this case insecurity regarding the client and our apparent lack of initial progress—the insecurity dissipates as it is held with love and a sense that nothing in particular needs to be done about it.

This process of acceptance parallels what occurs in meditation. Countless times thoughts and feelings arise. The ideal is to address them not through grasping or through getting seduced by their power, nor through brusquely pushing them away or running from them in a state of aversion; instead the mediator witnesses the thoughts or feelings, sees them for what they are, and in a state of equanimity returns to the breath. A discussion on mindfulness follows in the next chapter.

## RADICAL ACCEPTANCE IS NOT A DISTRACTION

As you read this discussion, you may question whether it is possible to devote this level of attention to process while simultaneously tracking the client's often complex story and crafting interventions. A few things are important to say in this regard. First, as you tune into what it takes to maintain a field of radical acceptance, you are doing *the work*. Again, the dualistic notion that there is mindful breathing or clinical process on the one hand and the real work of assessment and intervention on the other provides an artificial conceptual divide regarding what is important for clients. As we radically accept our clients, we validate them for who they are. They become more honest because they do not have to pretend they are someone else; they feel less shame; they feel like they deserve to occupy space on the planet. Attention and effort devoted to a radically accepting stance is well worth it and should not be divorced from your thinking about "intervening with clients."

Second, as we radically accept our clients as well as ourselves in the course of our work, strategies of change and implementation ideas are more likely to emerge from a mutual process of discovery. Clients are more likely to experience that the practitioner is working *with* them rather than doing something *to* them. Clients have the space to internalize insights and develop personal strategies rather than have interpretations and change plans imposed upon them. The practitioner's emphasis on creating a space of radical acceptance, therefore, lessens the need for the practitioner to personally create and spit out brilliant plans and professional pronouncements. As we accept the wisdom of our clients and the sacredness of the environment, and remain open to our own ego demands and internal dialog, we are less likely to be reactive. In this state of nonreactivity, we are less likely to psychically flee from or fight with unpleasant thoughts or client mannerisms.

Radical acceptance of our clients, ourselves, and the client-practitioner field *as it is* slows the session down and enhances practitioner and client clarity. Michael Jordan described this slowing down when he was interviewed about his game-winning shot for the Chicago Bulls' sixth championship. Though the hostile Utah crowd was screaming and collectively willing that he miss the last-second shot, though the time was winding down and all Utah Jazz players knew that he would put the fate of his team on his shoulders, Michael Jordan serenely took it all in. The world moved slowly for him in these moments, and he credited Phil Jackson's Zen approach for the way he was accepting the moment and tuning into the circumstances. There was a degree of effortlessness for him as he dribbled down the court, took note of nearby defenders and teammates, noticed the time clock and basket, made some evasive moves, and elevated his body and sank the shot.

Similarly with clients, our acceptance of the issues immediately relevant to the helping context—the ground of thoughts and feelings in the room as well as the possibilities for client well-being—are all present. Our tuning into reality as it is does not detract us from our work with clients. Our tuning in contributes to our soft front, our ability to let go, and our deeper connection with clients and with the task at hand.

## CONTEMPLATION EXERCISE

Let yourself breathe and drop any definitions that you may have of your client. Let your heart expand and find the space in your being to include this individual. Notice the universal nature of our masks—our roles, patterns of behavior, ways of coping, feelings, and stories. Notice how this strange and immensely powerful force that we call love creates the healthy container for our lives, gives us a sense that life is worth living and connects us to the bigger picture. Notice what it feels like when you put love and acceptance at the center of your relationships with clients.

This level of acceptance provides a fertile ground and valuable moisture for clients to grow even if their seeds related to health have hardly been watered their entire lives. After years of living in near-drought conditions in New Mexico, Joan Halifax conceded that she was beginning to lose faith in the proclamations of longtime residents who asserted that various flowers had blossomed in the area—flowers that she had not seen in her 15 years of living there. Finally, in the spring of 2005, the heavy winter's rain and snow-melt brought an array of beautiful wildflowers that she had never seen in the high desert valley. The dried seed beds made her think of the many human beings in the world who are themselves dried seed beds waiting to be watered. Radical acceptance of our clients and ourselves prepares the ground for these extremely dry and dormant seeds to flower.

## BRINGING IT HOME: PRINCIPLES OF RADICAL ACCEPTANCE IN A TEEN GROUP SETTING

Radical acceptance in a group setting refers to the social worker's profoundly embracing and opening his or her heart to the reality, behavior, feelings, story, and humanness of the group members as well as to the group's process (see Hayes, Follette, & Linehan, 2004). The social worker practicing radical acceptance maintains moment-to-moment awareness and equanimity and does not seek or crave for the group or its members to be any different than they are. Whether I am leading groups of diverse teens, dual-diagnosed addicts, disabled younger children, or mental health clinicians, I focus on facilitating and nurturing a group culture of radical acceptance. I have seen how this kind of environment contributes to high levels of intimate sharing, mutual respect, and positive outcomes. In one particular school-based group of seven high school boys (two African Americans, three Caucasians, one Latino, and one recently arrived Russian immigrant), members consistently told revealing personal stories. The radical acceptance environment seemed to have the following impacts in facilitating outcomes that the boys reported in individual de-briefing interviews: (a) it helped the diverse group members form a cohesive whole; (b) it created a powerful sense of universality which, in essence, was about each participant seeing and accepting his own and other group members' stories; (c) it allowed for expression of taboo feelings and dilemmas; (d) it normalized family difficulties; (e) it led to honest discussion regarding drug use as well as eventual plans to curtail such use; (f) it provided a forum to receive compliments (one member at the conclusion of the group commented, "Wow, I actually had something nice said to me"); (g) it provided opportunities for members to listen to each other and experience being listened to (one member reflected in the debriefing interview on his joy on hearing other group members talk—"I thought this is great . . . these douchebags are *talking* now"); (h) it established the ground for a caring, risk-taking environment. Members reported that at the conclusion of the group they felt closer to the group members and were friendly with them during the school day. Despite initial apprehensions about some of the group members, participants reported that earlier divisions melted away. Months after the conclusion of the group, the boys consistently asked me about starting up another boys' group (which I did undertake).

Radical acceptance refers to embracing, with an open heart, all that life presents. Radical acceptance incorporates, yet goes beyond, the Rogerian perspectives of positive regard and nonjudgmentalism toward individual clients and includes acceptance of the social worker's own here-and-now experience and process. Thus, radical acceptance has particular relevance for the group worker. When one radically accepts life as it is, one may comfortably sit in the midst of uncertainty—so common to group settings—and not panic and not react in order to re-assert control. When practicing radical acceptance, leaders are less likely to experience that their egos are on the line and are less likely to stifle creativity. In the midst of radical acceptance, the worker may witness when his or her mind is inclined toward unproductive thoughts, feeling states, and behavior and may invoke a self-compassionate message such as: "There I go trying to control things again."

Radical acceptance is about complete respect and understanding for people's lives and how their lives are manifested in terms of personal behavior. Those who experience a sense of radical acceptance toward the world as it is are likely to enjoy a bodily experience of relaxing with whatever arises, and even when not relaxing can, on some level, relax with how much they are not relaxing. In a state of radical acceptance, we become open to our own process of turmoil, anger, or inadequacy, and thus present a nondefended self to our clients. Even in the midst of a chaotic group session, the leader's self-message as well as the message to our clients is "thank-you" for the way things are.

Our open-heartedness means that we do not suffer as persistently from the constriction of fear. We try to remain open to the possibility of losing control as well as to the possibility that our openness leaves us vulnerable. At times, cofacilitator Kristin Love and I were open-hearted regarding our own fear and, because of our lack of physical or emotional constriction as well as our ability to see mental ruminations for what they were, we could sometimes transcend a flight-or-fight response regarding the group's process.

In terms of the process of the particular boys' group, part of our plan in building trust was to discuss, during our norm-building session, whether Kristin (an MSW intern at the time) should, as a female, co-lead the boys' group. Our openness to the boys' suspiciousness and reluctance, as well as our sincere, respectful, and humorous orientation to issues regarding a "female presence" helped set the tone for the group and for the way that other group members eventually treated each other.

Radical acceptance during this discussion as well as others meant that we embraced and validated the boys for their perspectives and stories as well as for their willingness and courage to mutually share their feelings and thoughts.

Radical acceptance provided a safe container for the co-construction, exploration, and subtle challenges to the adolescents' stories and ideas. Group-member involvement and participation were treated as sacred events, even while some of the group members were standing up and eating potato chips in the midst of another person's difficult story. We believed that the allowance for eating chips and joking set the tone for what Malekoff (2004) described as "welcoming the whole person, not just the troubled parts" (p. 39).

When one group member emphatically challenged the group and its leaders with "this group sucks" during the fourth session, the leaders' radical acceptance posture played a role in the eventual success of the group. The boy who made this statement, upon the group's conclusion, reflected to me his surprise about how I handled his outburst: "I thought to myself, he's not yelling at me yet. After this [situation], you showed me you weren't utterly and completely incompetent."

Another youth reflected on this same incident in a postgroup interview: "After [that boy] said that and you dealt with it, I thought this [the group] could be real cool."

The nature of the leaders' responses emerged from our nonreactivity as well as our willingness to see that the open expression of dissatisfaction actually represented group member strength. Radical acceptance served as a foundation for us to see member strengths and resilience in the midst of anger and turmoil and to abandon attachment to a particular adult-inspired outcome for that group session (completion of an exercise that we had prepared).

## RADICAL ACCEPTANCE AND CHANGE

Dialectical behavior therapy (DBT) has done a beautiful job in recent years of depicting the primary contradiction inherent in the therapy process. Clients come to helping practitioners because they are hurting, suffering, or acting destructively in some manner. Our fundamental charge whether arising from the clients directly or from the exhausted, overwhelmed, worried, or threatened referral source is to *create change* so that client pain and suffering is reduced and behavior is less erratic, destructive, or frightening. When change occurs to everyone's satisfaction, people receiving therapy may: (a) feel more competent in the world and better about themselves; (b) be less prone to having waves of despair, anger, and fear rip them from their moorings and sweep them into turbulent seas of demons and unpredictability; or (c) find themselves in trouble less frequently. People around adolescents who are beneficiaries of therapeutic change worry less about an impending crisis or a volatile or violent emotional display and the youth themselves may have fewer visits to principals' offices, police stations, and emergency rooms. Creating client change seems to promise not only these absolutely precious goodies, but also can make everybody (our teen clients and their desperate family members, teachers, classmates, friends, and neighbors) happier.

Despite the apparent promise of therapeutic change, clients—and teens in particular—rarely seem to engage with an individual practitioner or group leader on personal change agendas, regardless of the degree to which they are suffering. In fact, DBT grew out of the founders' observations that "the unrelenting focus on change inherent to cognitive behavior therapy was invalidating" (Sanderson, 2003, p. 1). Clients want their group and individual practitioners and therapists to accept them and engage with them on the level of who they are, what they think, how they feel, and what their story is. In the case of teens, they are particularly tuned into whether professional helpers are fundamentally accepting or more interested in molding them to conform to an adult image of success. The less accepting adult not only hyperfocuses on getting youth to change, but she or he is more inclined to be dismissive of youth dilemmas or perspectives and label or categorize youth as either underachieving, conduct-disordered, delinquent, drama-queen, thug, depressed, drug addict, and some other negative descriptor.

Practitioner over-investment in agenda-setting and implicit or explicit nonacceptance may be layered on the self-denigration, personal insecurity, and profound feelings of unworthiness that struggling teens experience even before they enter some kind of helping relationship. Teenage thoughts of being damaged goods, incapable of success and unworthy of taking up space on the planet, must therefore be ameliorated with acceptance-based strategies and not always with cognitive ones that—in my experience with adolescents—sometimes contain the implicit message that the teens were stupid for having some of the thoughts they had about themselves and the world.

As we look closely at the value of acceptance-based strategies, we see that they not only relate to providing a foundation for client change and a container for client risk-taking, they contribute directly to a desirable outcome: enhanced client acceptance. These strategies not only assist the social worker or counselor in building effective, trusting, and validating therapeutic relationships that are the necessary foundation for pursuing the difficult, vulnerable work of behavioral and emotional change, but self-acceptance becomes a major life skill for clients to acquire, helping them pursue the path of what Marsha Linehan calls "a life worth living."

## RADICAL ACCEPTANCE IS NOT FOR WIMPS

On the surface, radical acceptance can appear to be a philosophy extolling the virtues of docility, nonassertiveness, and in-action. Groups of people who historically have been oppressed may understandably be suspicious of its principles, and practitioners recognizing the need for structure, boundaries, and limits may be wary that a radical acceptance style leads one to be an ineffective doormat. I would argue that, in fact, radical acceptance does not incline one toward docility or weakness. Instead, people approaching individuals or situations from a stance of radical acceptance are inclined to see and accept things as they are and often become more prepared—with a strong back—to respond. Accepting things as they are does not mean *approval* or sanctioning for outlandish, oppressive, or self-defeating behavior. Accepting things as they are means coming face-to-face with the reality that countless moments and circumstances have led up to this very moment and no degree of denial, aggressiveness, wishing it were different, or mental bargaining is going to make things as you would like them to be. In the midst of a slow, deliberate breath, one experiences the total realization or acceptance that—*yes*—*this is happening.* In this moment, the individual essentially becomes one with the experience because there is no resistance to what is unfolding.

In contrast to openly facing or accepting reality, a woman, for example, who is being abused by her partner may engage in thinking such as: "This is not really happening" or "If I had just acted differently, this nightmare would not occur." Opening to the reality of what is happening—radically accepting the reality—would more likely lead, for this individual, to more effective responses. This example illustrates why radical acceptance should not be equated with passivity.

In addition to bargaining or denial, the *non*practice of radical acceptance leads to conflict-oriented (fight) or aversive/denial (flight) strategies. Radical acceptance allowed me to sit with the feelings of incompetence, the fears of losing control, the vulnerabilities and embarrassments related to looking bad in front of my intern, and the thought that the expression of "this group sucks" would undermine whatever progress the group had been making to that point. Rigorous honesty concerning the situation as well as this situation's or my own dark side allowed me to respond effectively from a place of strength, nondefensiveness, and compassion. Rather than ignore the comment (flight or freeze), blame the participant for his lack of constructive involvement (fight), take on the whole group for its negative attitude (fight), "therapeutically" turn the comment into a clever inquiry tying the participant's disappointment with prior events in his life (flight/fight), or sink into hopelessness and despair (flight), it was important to radically accept the comment and all that led up to it with equanimity and an open heart. Seeing the truth in this manner does not suggest any particular action or inaction per se. What it does suggest is the greater likelihood of a response that is compassionate and skillful because responses will arise from a courageous face-to-face encounter with what is.

Finally, radical acceptance is not about dismissing rules or structures or approaching life or situations with a laissez-faire, anything-goes philosophy. In order for group clients, particularly adolescents, to take risks, it is necessary to establish some sense of a holding environment or therapeutic container. As helping practitioners, we need to create a validating environment that not only helps affirm our clients, but also where our clients feel some degree of safety. Calling a gathering of individuals "a group" is not adequate for establishing a container of radical acceptance, self-affirmation, growth, honest examination, risk-taking, and mutual support. Structure, boundaries, and norms are essential components for constructing the container. Thus, the radically accepting practitioner does not eschew structure nor does she or he become a punching bag. The radically accepting practitioner embraces the apparent contradiction or dialectic regarding structure and rules on the one hand versus spontaneity and freedom on the other.

## RADICAL ACCEPTANCE AND MARGINALIZED STATUS OF CLIENTS

It is so easy to see many of our clients as a lost lot, so badly in need of our educated direction as well as in need of a dose of our version of reality. Many people we work with seem overly confused, aggressive, poor, dirty, violent, depressed, despairing, hopeless, impulsive, and hurting. Our time to work with these "sorry folks"—as some may view our clients—is limited, and at the same time our work setting's demands for documentation and concrete outcomes is intense. These kinds of dynamics seem conducive to quickly imposing our wise, educated, more sane and stable views on our clients whose lives seem to be littered with failure and ineptitude.

How do we work from a space of radical acceptance when confronted with these realities? Part of our stance involves the recognition that embracing or accepting the client-worker space involves embracing the entire context associated with the client and the worker. Thus, I radically accept that all the clients whom I see in a dual-diagnosis, substance abuse group are subject to consistent urine tests before they arrive at group. I see that they are highly attuned to whether they are "advancing" in the program. I see their courage and sincerity as they claim that they do not want to do drugs; I know their stories of betrayal and profound pain: how their family members have betrayed them, how they have betrayed their family members and themselves, how life has not turned out as they would have wished. I try to hold it all as I sit in the group with these wonderful human beings.

One intense issue raised during the weekly process group (the two other weekly groups are educational) took one-half of the group's one and a half hours. I told myself that this issue was everyone's issue, so all would benefit. However, only 45 minutes remained for eight or nine other group members to check-in. The issue I decided to focus on involved one group member: Maria's expression of irritation toward another group member, John. Maria discussed how during her advancement ceremony the week before, John motioned to one of the group facilitators that he wanted to see the facilitator outside the group for a moment. Maria developed an entire story in her mind that during this momentary meeting, John was accusing her of absences or some kind of rule infraction. Maria became angry, not only at John's brief whispering to the facilitator but also at the accusations she imagined were contained in John's message. John, on the other hand, revealed that he did not at all try to undermine Maria's group advancement ceremony. He believed that he was very considerate of Maria because under most conditions he would have exploded during her graduation because her advancement made him feel so hurt about his own long struggle to advance. John faced Maria and said (with apparent sincerity), "I handled it the best I could. . . . I did not want to take away from your day; I was happy for you. . . . I never said anything negative about your advancing" (which the group leader corroborated).

Maria, however, was not so forgiving. She repeatedly scolded John for bringing attention to himself during her moment to shine. The group members were kind with Maria but could also see John's sincerity and knew that he *had* made great progress in his avoidance of a major scene. One could sense the disgust of the social work intern as well as some group members with Maria's inflexible stance. In the midst of it all, I radically accepted the positions, the hardness, the softness, the apparent reasonableness, the apparent unreasonableness, the unspoken, the reactivity, and the unknown of all that was happening.

I saw myself taking a few steps down the analytical and judgmental path. In other words, I asked myself whether Maria was so sensitive about John's actions because she had, in fact, gotten away with some rule infraction and whether John—despite his denial—was being his narcissistic self and with some degree of intention was raining on Maria's parade. I quickly let go of these fleeting "professional judgments" or clever analyses. I sensed that they would do little good here as Maria and John struggled and stumbled through the pain of their now-conflicted relationship and the group struggled through their pain and through their sense of helplessness about how to help them. Radically accepting the moment allowed me to watch the arising professional story about how each one's respective deficiencies created the difficulties the entire group found itself in. If I had chosen this direction, I would have steered clear of the vulnerability that I, myself, experienced when I eventually plunged into the pain and mess that was taking place in the room that day.

Plunging into the pain and mess meant that I experienced a sense of incompetence as the group leader. This dynamic was enhanced because the well-loved and respected coleader was phasing out of the group and because the interns were not ready to assume a major responsibility for group leadership—they were supposed to be learning group leadership from me. There did not seem to be any way out; tears and distress were increasing. I sensed that the scenario touched deep wounds of personal betrayal that the group would not be able to contain at this point, nor was there enough time for this kind of exploration. In the midst of deep uncertainty, I decided to focus on Maria's and John's listening to and hearing the other. I was firm about slowing the process down and not allowing reactive responses. Other group members gave feedback, particularly to Maria, that was insightful. I framed Maria's and John's exchange as well as the group member feedback in two broad areas. First, I discussed how Maria and John were particularly courageous in how they processed this experience, and I normalized their exchange. The exchange during this particular group and the conflict of the past week took place, I said, because of our human imperfections that come up as we deal with situations that affect our emotions. For different reasons, advancement was an emotional time for Maria and John. John's hurt feelings started leaking out and the manner in which he attempted to deal with them led Maria to have her feelings leak out. When the group container has two people leaking at once, the group feels like it is going to get flooded. People do leak, groups do feel overwhelmed, of course, this happens.

Second, I discussed how hard it must be to be an agency client because the agency is always evaluating their progress, insisting on a rigid code of conduct, conducting drug testing, and helping to determine whether their involvement in the program merits their continued freedom from jail and/or their ability to raise their children vis-à-vis Child Protective Services. The issue of advancement (and rejection or delay of advancement) is highly emotional. Although many clients are sincerely and deeply grateful for the role that the agency has played in their lives, there frequently seems to be shame for the manner in which the individual was referred to the program and the manner in which the client is forced to continue treatment. Additionally, of course, many clients were raised by addicts themselves who did not always tune into their achievements or immediate needs. For these reasons, I surmised, the whole question of advancement is an emotionally loaded issue for many. In the midst of "it all," Maria and John were doing a beautiful job of dealing with what happened. It was not neat, and one man noted how the process crept along at a snail's pace; however, the work was positive and valuable.

There was group recognition of these issues. Maria and John softened and admitted that each one could have handled the situation differently. In order to reach this point in the group, I needed to accept that someone's individual work would probably be compromised that day, and, more importantly, accept that there was a risk to revealing the group members' anger, disappointment, confusion, and pain. As mentioned, I had been informed of this conflict before the group started that day. I needed to accept the part of me that wanted to brush the conflict under the rug or to "just see" if it would come up. Throughout the work, I accepted the uncertainty of the entire enterprise. At times, I noticed myself tightening and wishing the group could somehow move on; then I would accept my wish to escape the ambiguity and attempt to center myself in the midst of the uncertain swamp.

Interestingly, the interns did not appreciate the uncertainty. One mentioned how frustrated she was with Maria's unwillingness to hear where John was coming from. I could sense my impatience arise in response to her impatience; I inwardly smiled at my response and calmly said that her feelings were completely understandable. Our job, though, is to remain open-hearted to the experiences of others rather than reactive — as much as possible. I am a believer in parallel process and as such would rather model acceptance of my intern's perspective than lecture her about her need to be less judgmental and more accepting.

## PATIENCE, GIVING, AND RADICAL ACCEPTANCE

Our commitment to being patient facilitates the nonreactivity we wish to generate to maintain a field of radical acceptance. Often patience refers to a willingness to wait until the desired outcome finally occurs, like tolerating a long grocery checkout line. The patience referred to here, however, involves the practitioner as a serene witness who does not "bite the bullet" while waiting for a self-designed outcome, but instead involves a quality of patience that embraces the uncertainty of the journey as well as the fallibilities of self and other. Patience is one of the highest gifts that we can give to ourselves and to our clients. As Zen Master Suzuki Roshi once said to his students, "You are all perfect beings, the only thing that you need is a little work." Our patience comes from the deep recognition that we all, in fact, are perfect beings. Our mistakes (large and small), our destructive behaviors and thoughts, our barriers (real and imagined) make up the fabric of our lives and our life stories. None of these elements are permanent; thus, change occurs in all of these realms. Our patience regarding our client's fallibilities, the snail's pace at which change occurs, and the degree to which clients and community members do not embrace us are all met with compassionate patience.

Your ability as a practitioner to be patient vitally contributes to the radical acceptance you may generate. In a society that clamors for immediate gratification and is quick to label individuals as nonproductive or losers, being patient and teaching the skill of patience is invaluable for our clients. Significant periods of staying clean from drugs accumulate one day at a time, positive friendships for disabled youth develop slowly, stable employment is difficult to attain, a reduction in long-standing depression or anxiety or pervasive hallucinations may take months, rigid behavior patterns and lapses into negative thinking or feeling states may persist. Your patience with your clients (as well as yourself) translates to the client's self-patience. Patience is a key ingredient in constructing the radical acceptance atmosphere.

Should patience not serve as a foundation for work, we end up directly or indirectly berating our clients for their failure to measure up to our own image. We become irritated with our clients in the same way we may become irritated with the checkout line customer who waits to figure out whether to pay with cash, ATM, or credit until *after* the groceries have all been scanned. As irritation gives way to anger, we may conjure up stories regarding reasons for the inconsiderate behavior of that customer. Is he too narcissistic to realize that his behavior affects others who are waiting? Just what is his problem?

Jack Kornfield, a well-known Buddhist psychologist, tells a wonderful story about a man who had served in the military and was taking a meditation–stress reduction class. He found himself standing in a checkout line behind a woman who was holding a baby and only one grocery item. Strangely, she bypassed the express line. When she approached the register, she lifted the baby up and let a doting cashier hold it. The woman with the one grocery item, the cashier, and the baby began an extensive three-way interaction. Meanwhile, the stress reduction student was becoming increasingly annoyed.

He was prone to impatience and he—perhaps thanks to the stress reduction class—became aware of tensing up, of feeling progressively more angry, and of attributing judgments to the women regarding their selfishness.

Based on the class lesson that he had just received, he started to breathe more softly and deliberately and relax. He even shifted his attention to the baby and noticed its appearance. When he finally arrived at the cashier, he commented on how cute the baby was. The cashier thanked him and told him how wonderful it was that she could see *her baby* a few moments during her working day. "My husband was in the Air Force and he died last year in a plane crash," she said. "Now my mother brings the baby in so I can see him for a few minutes during my working day."

## CONTEMPLATION EXERCISE

Do you know how much your patience means to your clients? Please be still and contemplate this question. How does your radical acceptance of your client, the context, and yourself set the ground for the kind of strong back and soft front work that we intend to do?

In the next chapter, we discuss methods for cultivating practitioner mindfulness that generate radical acceptance.

**Chapter Four**

# MINDFULNESS: STEADYING THE MIND AND BEING PRESENT

*Beyond Empathy Skills and Counter-Transference*

*It only takes a reminder to breathe,
a moment to be still, and just like that,
something in me settles, softens, makes
space for imperfection. The harsh voice
of judgment drops to a whisper and I
remember again that life isn't a relay
race; that we will all cross the finish
line; that waking up to life is what we
were born for. As many times as I
forget, catch myself charging forward
without even knowing where I'm going,
that many times I can make the choice
to stop, to breathe, and be, and walk
slowly into the mystery.*

**—Danna Faulds**

Mindfulness fuels our ability to maintain radical acceptance of ourselves and our clients and steadies the mind in order that we meet the present moment. Marsha Linehan (2003) described mindfulness as the light that we need when we are trying to walk through a living room crowded with furniture.

47

When we are able to clearly see what is in front of us and around us, we are able to navigate our way successfully. On the other hand, when our mind is not so settled, we are inclined to become seduced by passing wishes or fantasies or distracted by on-coming feelings, thoughts, or moods. We bump into the furniture with our unsettled mind and we may start to indulge in wishes that our client be other than who she or he is. Habitual thought patterns — even if they lead to ineffective responses or bring suffering — may toss us about in the absence of mindfulness. For the purposes of this chapter, mindfulness refers to: (a) the practitioner's focused concentration in a primary activity (e.g., breathing or listening to a client); (b) the practitioner's ability to witness arising thoughts, feelings, and activity without becoming highly distracted; and (c) the practitioner's equanimity while being with whatever arises.

Zen Priest Reb Anderson's basic meditation instruction is to relax with whatever arises. This kind of teaching represents the essence of radical acceptance. Notice what arises in the mind, do not run toward it, do not run away from it, do not freeze and become enamored or fixated . . . just relax and return to the breath.

Even as you notice how unsettled your mind actually becomes, relax with the unsettled mind and return to the breath. When we are able to relax with, we are able to *"be with."* We sit down with our clients — *as they are* — and open our hearts to their lives. At the same time, the simple effort directed toward focusing our attention on the breath — a concentration practice — assists our being single-minded and present for our clients. Our clients not only need our open, radical acceptance, they also require that we set a structure for the relationship and focus on what may be helpful. (Mindfulness exercises are offered later in the chapter that can facilitate your acquisition of these skills.)

Some life and client situations create favorable conditions for having an unsettled mind. One such example occurred when a social worker discussed his frustrations regarding a client who consistently called his cell phone regarding issues that did not seem to meet the threshold for an "appropriate" call. (Being on-call was a component of this social worker's program.) The practitioner described that, as his client's phone calls continued, his reactions progressively intensified from irritation to significant frustration to self-righteous rage. His strategy for dealing with his intense feelings was to suppress his anger as much as possible, to talk to the client about feeling frustrated with the client's continual calling, and to vent his outrage in the supervision group. This pattern of suppression and ventilation ran counter to mindfulness-based acceptance. While the client was in the practitioner's presence, the practitioner was lost in a story that involved the client's pathology, the practitioner's victimization at the hands of the client, and the practitioner's doomsday prediction that whatever happened in this case was likely not to be positive.

In general, the practitioner who feels reactive and then decides to suppress the reactivity is spending an inordinate amount of energy and attention on his or her own cyclical process. Ironically, despite the energy that is expended, little relief is obtained. The practitioner continues to fight the endless battle of keeping grinding resentment, doubt, and despair at bay. As this battle intersects with the practitioner's pathologizing the client and with a growing sense of personal victimization, she or he barely registers and connects with the *client's* real life challenges and pain.

As I sat and listened to the social worker's dilemma, I noticed that I became impatient with *the practitioner's* level of impatience. In a manner similar to how he likely loses contact with his client, I lost contact with the social worker's suffering. This kind of parallel process is uncanny in supervision arrangements. In the course of a supervisee's telling stories of his or her work with clients, it is quite common for me to experience the similar field that exists when the supervisee actually sits with the client.

I was mindful of my intentions, my tone of voice, my thoughts, and my feelings as I addressed the social worker. I was also aware of his expression and the group energy in the room. I was mindful of my own irritation; then, I tried to *transform* the irritation to both a feeling of kindness and generosity for the practitioner and a deep intention to say something that would be helpful for the practitioner and for his work with the client. Transformation occurs when we make a conscious attempt to shift a feeling state or a pattern of thinking. If we are mindful of our anger, for example, we can breathe through the experience, realize that it is impermanent, and attempt to replace this experience with a mindful and open-hearted expression of compassion, understanding, or caring. Thich Nhat Hanh (2001) discusses how mindfulness can transform the compost of anger into a compassionate response:

> You need to sustain your mindfulness for a certain amount of time in order for the flower of anger to open herself. . . . Your anger is very difficult to enjoy, but if you know how to take care of it, to cook it, then the negative energy of your anger will become the positive energy of understanding and compassion. (p. 29)

The mindful awareness of our anger or annoyance is the necessary first step. Without this kind of awareness, we are less capable of working with our emotions and less likely to fully appreciate how ever-changing and whimsical our emotions and thoughts are. Breathing slowly and mindfully diminishes the hot flame of our inflammatory thoughts and feelings; they become less solid and easier to touch. If we do not attend to our thoughts and feelings, we are more likely to stay angry or annoyed and may even use labels in a self-righteous and dismissive manner. We attend to our thoughts and feelings with compassionate awareness.

## ZEN AND MINDFULNESS

It may be worth mentioning that there are different perspectives concerning the relationship between Zen and mindfulness practice. Zen monk Thich Nhat Hanh advances mindfulness as a core practice for healthy individuals and for a healthy planet. In one of his first published books, *The Miracle of Mindfulness*, he discusses how important it is to mindfully engage in our daily activities:

> If while washing the dishes, we think only of the cup of tea that awaits us, thus hurrying to get the dishes out of the way as if they were a nuisance, then we are not "washing the dishes to wash the dishes." What's more, we are not alive during the time we are washing the dishes. In fact we are completely incapable of realizing the miracle of life while standing at the sink. If we can't wash the dishes, the chances are we won't be able to drink our tea either. . . . Thus . . . we are incapable of actually living one minute of life. (1987, pp. 4–5)

Ultimately, Nhat Hanh believes that residing in mindfulness is the core of a joyful and peaceful life. On the other hand, if we are unaware while engaging in an activity or disconnected while encountering people, then we are missing our appointment with life. Connection to the present moment allows us to touch the sacredness of all things and to cherish our moment-to-moment life.

Ethical and skillful behavior flows from mindfulness. As a result, Thich Nhat Hanh (1993) has framed Buddhist moral precepts as *mindfulness trainings* and has attempted to broaden the application of mindfulness beyond Buddhist cultural and religious roots.

When Thich Nhat Hanh begins meditation instruction with a Zen-like singular focus on the breath, he envisions this work as *mindfully* watching and being with the breath. The ability to bring focus and concentrated awareness to the breath itself inevitably exercises the mind for engaging in mindful attention.

It is confusing that mindfulness practice is often equated with insight meditation or *Vipassana*. In Vipassana, the meditator applies mental notes to the waves of mental or emotional states that pass through the consciousness. In the midst of a grinding internal dialog about how you failed with a particular client, you may apply a note or label "self-judgment" before you return to the breath. Gently applying the note "self-judgment" may decrease the emotional turmoil and help you disembark from the train that carries you *and* the mental/emotional activity that is invested in the failure narrative. From a Vipassana perspective, you may be more prepared *to drop the distracting and unhelpful story* because it is packaged up into a little box marked "self-judgment." The story's details disintegrate as you see the package for what it is—a passing cloud of thinking activity.

Unlike Thich Nhat Hanh, some Buddhists make a strong distinction between the mindfulness (Vipassana) practice just described and concentration practice. In Zen, the emphasis tends to be on developing concentration or achieving *Samadhi*—a state of intense absorption where one is ". . . totally committed—almost *held* . . . —within one attentional field to the exclusion of others" (Austin, 1998, p. 474). Life from this vantage point is said to "flow joyously."

Many Zen Masters believe that developing concentration is an important base because the mind is often so scattered and deluded. It was my personal experience that labeling thoughts played into my already overly entertained, distracted, and intellectualized mind. I appreciated the simplicity of the Zen approach and the bare bones instructions of "watching the breath." This simple practice clears the field and creates conditions for enhanced mindfulness.

Thus, there is a degree of ambiguity about the term *mindfulness*. Some, like Thich Nhat Hanh, emphasize the boundlessness (nonseparateness) of mindfulness and concentration. For the purposes of this book, we speak of mindfulness in these kind of inclusive terms. Our beginning point will be to enhance our commitment to be within one "attentional field":

> Whatever names attach to Buddhist mindfulness, it still starts out the same way: as a *nonreactive, bare awareness open to any-thing*. . . . "All" you must do is set aside mental space, then

dedicate it fully to the here and now. . . . (We are aiming toward having capacities to) . . . register the bare perception, observe with detachment, notice without elaboration. After a long while, the brain finally seems emptied of all save the first, fresh entry of raw sensory data and that open, mirror-like receptivity which greets it. (Austin, 1998, pp. 126–127)

I have found that helping practitioners who begin to tune into their breath experience benefit from enhanced mindfulness. We proceed in this simple fashion.

## MINDFULNESS AND THE BREATH

Awareness of our breath returns us to our body and to the rhythms of the universe. Our typical state of affairs is to be lost in our thoughts—ruminating about plans for the future, replaying past events, and judging the value and worthiness of ourselves and others. We chase after or seek to possess people or things that we have judged to be pleasant and we try to stay away from or shed that which we have judged to be unpleasant. We spend so much time playing the tapes and movies about who we are, what we want, and how we will acquire things, people, or status that we become accustomed to our mind's ability to occupy or entertain us. Joan Halifax uses the metaphor of our mind as the entertainment center. This metaphor refers to the pre-Internet and iPod age when the centerpiece of many living rooms was a monstrously large piece of furniture that held a television, turntable (which played things called "records"), tape player, the family record and tape collections, an amplifier which incorporated a radio, and large speakers— sometimes as many as four. Not only was the entertainment center a cacophony of sound and imposing machinery, the sheer number of large knobs and brightly lit dials and meters added other elements of interest. I have memories of holding my 2-year-old son and walking past our family's version of the entertainment center. The knobs and buttons called out for him to touch them and roll them around his fingers whenever they were within reach. Now we carry our entertainment centers with us in the form of cell phones and MP3 players.

When we are aware of our breath, the entertainment center loses its grip. We sense that we are grounded and experience peace and acceptance. Not only do the noise and stimulation from the entertainment center arise and fade away, emotions and thoughts that cause personal suffering and that are fueled by a ruminating and worried mind also diminish.

As we tune into our breathing, the power and overwhelming nature of our different stories lessens because we see the narratives for what they are — stories. We sense that there is more to us than the trauma that we have suffered, the negative ideas we have about ourselves, the difficult events that are weighing on us, the fears we have about the future, and the critical things that people have said to us. All of these elements are no longer solid truths that burden our existence but are passing waves of thoughts and feelings that are archetypes of the human condition.

Our breath is the path embodying the essence of our being. Williams, Teasdale, Segal, and Kabat-Zinn (2007) writing on the benefits of mindfulness for the treatment of depression do an excellent job of describing the potential of the mindful awareness of the breath:

> [W]e could say that stress, fatigue, and afflictive emotions thrive in the absence of the *fresh air of awareness*. It is not that, with awareness, they cease to exist, but that awareness puts more space around them, and such spaciousness, like fresh air to the spores (spores are a metaphor of negative feeling states or thoughts which rely upon the absence of oxygen) provides an environment in which the self-diminishing and constricting frames of mind no longer thrive. Mindfulness detects them early on, sees them clearly, and notices how they arise and can pass away. It offers us a way of seeing clearly without having to get caught in them. We don't usually inhabit or even visit this dimension of our own minds. . . . Although it is a powerful capacity we all have, we mostly ignore it. (p. 71, italics mine)

Mindfulness thus brings stability to the mind and an internal confidence that we can maintain a strong back in the face of turmoil and strife. With troublesome or invasive feelings and thoughts, we observe them as frames of mind that will eventually pass or be transformed. As we become more anchored in our breath, we are less moved by our chaotic minds or by difficult and unpredictable circumstances. We become profoundly aware that our judgments of self and other are mere stories and that our feelings and thoughts are secretions of the mind.

One student commented on the role that mindfulness had in steadying her mind and helping her stay present at an intense community meeting:

> I noticed sudden feelings of nervousness during the conversation when my heart rate would begin to speed up and I would feel

anxious to argue my point. Because it would not have been effective to argue . . . I observed these internal feelings, and then attempted to leave them so that I could stay with the present conversation, rather than being drawn into my thoughts about nervous feelings.

It is beneficial for our direct service clients, as well, when we are able to experience the sense that whatever arises is workable. Workability here does not equate with a robotic and nonemotional way of being. Instead the breath anchors us in the experience so that we are able to meet whatever occurs. We may even have to deal with our sense of being overwhelmed and insecure. We know that with our breath we can meet these feelings. We may have to work with clients who are angry with us and who seem to be unaffected by our attempts to help. We can meet this situation and whatever thoughts or feelings arise in response. We may become scared while we are working with some people because they remind us of ourselves, of times when we were vulnerable, or because they just seem dangerous. We can meet this fear.

Ultimately, we can meet it all, including our own death and our fears about death. It is all workable. We learn to continue to ask ourselves the following questions: Should we lean toward the world of workability grounded in our calm, full breath or toward the world of despair and anxiety of the future while holding our breath? Which of these alternatives is healthier for ourselves and our clients? We address these questions with the full realization that we cannot just snap our fingers and suddenly live in a state of greater serenity. Some of us are wired for anxiety or, perhaps, we have suffered through events that have made our organisms reactive and vigilant. Some of us have strongly ingrained habits to indulge in judging mercilessly, perseverating about the past or future, or cooking up schemes related to controlling the uncontrollable. Regardless of our historical patterns or habits, we, at the very least, can contemplate that life lived in the present moment renders us less troubled and more available for others.

It is our calm sense of workability—anchored in the breath—that allows radical acceptance to be more than a mental approach to the world. We experience radical acceptance as a mind-body process that is integral to our strong back and soft front.

## BREATHING FOR PRACTITIONERS

Mindfulness has been touted for its potential applications to clients and client problems (Kabat-Zinn, 1990; Linehan, 2003; Williams et al., 2007). Marsha Linehan (2003) in particular understood mindfulness' potential in settling the mind and helping to create greater emotional stability. For this reason, she placed the cultivation of mindfulness as the central skill that clients labeled as borderline personality disordered needed to acquire. Her work with this clientele revealed that a roller-coaster emotional and cognitive life was responsible for inducing great suffering and episodes of emotional crisis. Practitioners are not immune to a roller coaster of emotions and thoughts in our own personal lives and certainly bear witness to the painful and distressing lives of our clients. The potential for mindfulness to contribute to practitioner well-being and effectiveness has to this point not been adequately emphasized.

Enhancing our capacity to calm our distracting voices, diminish our troubling or seductive thoughts, and enter situations with confidence about meeting the moment has enormous consequences for our clients. Our presence is the gift with which our clients first make contact. We offer them our presence through being awake in the present moment.

## MINDFULNESS 101: GETTING STARTED

Cultivating the breath as a foundation of mindfulness is not difficult. I have worked with students, clients, and practitioners who were not meditators and who experienced benefits from a minimal level of engagement with mindful breathing exercises. Students and practitioners have reported that as a result of mindful breathing, they have felt healthier overall and have experienced less reactivity and greater awareness with their clients. Various students have told me that as a result of their enhanced mindful attention, they were able to apply mindfulness in their social lives and were, thus, more able to tune into their partners' needs and communication. Some have reported being amazed after realizing how infrequently they had been truly present for their partners, children, family members, and friends.

You do not have to be in a meditation hall or get into a fancy posture to begin. It is best to sit straight in a chair and notice the feeling of your feet on the ground and the weight of your buttocks and thighs on the chair. (If sitting up fairly straight is challenging, you may lie down.) You may use these instructions as a guide to get you started individually, or a group or class leader may calmly and slowly recite them:

- Gently lower your gaze. You may close your eyes or keep them slightly open—whatever is more comfortable.
- Let your breathing slow down and begin to focus on how your breath moves throughout your body.

- Let your breath originate in your abdomen and notice how your abdomen expands and contracts. Embody the sense of strong back, soft front.
- As you inhale, be aware of "breathing in"; as you exhale, be aware of "breathing out."
- Continue this pattern for 10 breaths (a breath is an inhalation and exhalation).
- Slowly open your eyes.

Although this exercise appears to be simple, the results from steadily practicing it may be profound. There are a few important points that will assist you while you practice.

First, work on maintaining the spirit that *everything that happens* during the mindful breathing exercise is perfectly fine. Your mind may be distracted; you may spend most of the time planning, obsessing, or ruminating, or you may spend most of the time focused on your breath. When you have gone somewhere else, come back to your breath. As you come back, do so without any judgment. Coming back to your breath is an exercise in coming back to the present—it is valuable and worthy. Coming back to your breath over and over again is like coming back to your life or to your client over and over again. As you meet the present moment, welcome yourself back with kindness. This is more productive than beating yourself up for leaving your breath. If your mind has stayed away and you have been playing at the entertainment center, then the exercise of coming back after the extended absence is also a good exercise. If your mind has been with the breath, then you have had the experience of your mind staying with the breath and being present. This discussion reinforces the great Zen Master Dogen's assertion that there is no good or bad meditation experience.

Our comparing and judging mind is quite accustomed to evaluating our performance. We may even use our mind's attempts at passing judgment as an opportunity to observe. We learn to see the judging and comparing thoughts as passing clouds rather than as reality about the way things are. When we come back to our breath, we disarm thoughts relating to how well or how poorly we are doing. As these thoughts are increasingly seen for what they are—unhelpful, habitual, nontruthful secretions of mind—we develop the skill of focusing on an object of attention which is our breath. This skill translates to our work with clients. We develop the capacity to avoid getting caught in our fantasies, and we do not as readily mistake our judgments or descriptions of our clients for the client's reality. We enter the client's world calm and focused.

Second, start with a *modest level of engagement*. John Kabat-Zinn (1990) describes mindfulness as compassionate awareness. Be compassionate with yourself as you embark on this new path. You may repeat the exercise and continue with 10 breaths each day for a period of time. When you feel ready to attempt more you may choose to do mindfulness practice for 5 minutes a day. There is no particular destination here. You may become a regular meditator, or you may occasionally remember to take a few deep breaths before you begin a client session or before you meet with your supervisor. Notice whether you start becoming future-oriented about how much you are going to eventually meditate or what mindfulness courses you will eventually take, and so on. Also notice whether you beat yourself up regarding the days that you have not consciously practiced mindfulness or over the fact that you have decided that this mindful breathing stuff is not for you. We bring our own patterns of thinking to this endeavor. Maintain compassion for yourself regardless of the circumstances. You may become a wonderful helping practitioner without engaging in this practice, or you may find that another practice such as prayer or contemplating your personal intentions may make more sense for helping you wake up to the present moment.

Third, *cultivate self-compassion* during the mindfulness experiences themselves. You may experience that your mind seems highly distracted a good proportion of the time. Sometimes you may feel like quitting or you may become disgusted with yourself or with the process. Each time you return to your breath is an *opportunity* to cultivate self-compassion. Your familiar response may be to berate yourself for an inadequate performance as you return to your breath; you have the opportunity to be kind to yourself instead.

Finally, *appreciate the simplicity and profundity of your mind's capacity for concentration*. Zen Master Thich Nhat Hanh suggests that beginners follow their breath with the thoughts, "breathing in . . . breathing out." This approach may be helpful because the mind can be occupied with simple phrases and is somewhat less able to jump from branch to branch in the manner that Zen teachers describe as monkey mind. Awareness of breathing in/ awareness of breathing out or counting your breaths (in-out = 1; in-out = 2 . . .) may be a practice that you engage in for years. As we focus on our breath, we stop. We bring focused, calm awareness to the present moment and transcend society's pull to engage in reactive thinking and action. We eschew the refrain of "don't just sit there, do something," and instead adopt the mantra of "don't just do something, sit there." The mindful awareness of your breath is a foundation for connecting in the moment with our clients and with the world as it is and for dropping story lines, afflictive emotions, and other distractions. We engage in concentrated breathing not so we can endlessly sit and do nothing. *Our commitment is to engage* but to do so with thoughtfulness, nonreactivity, and open-heartedness. As Thich Nhat Hanh (2007) stated, "Imagine the power of our actions if each one contained one hundred percent of our attention" (p. 41).

## LETTING GO

The transformation of feeling states, as just discussed, is one strategy for dealing with emotions or thoughts that are unhelpful or potentially destructive. When immersed in irritation, resentment, despair, or anger, another approach for maintaining productive and helpful feeling states is *letting go*. Of course, letting go is often easier said than done, and there are many paths we may pursue to engage in the process. Letting go is a powerful act that may be practiced numerous times within a given day. While leading a letting-go group, I witnessed that participants focused their efforts at releasing destructive mind states, stories about others or themselves, material possessions, expectations of others, desires to control life events, preferences, and resentments. Group participants grew in their mindfulness and their appreciation of the multiple times throughout the day in which it was important to let go. As a result, members reported that they became more peaceful with themselves and their surroundings and more accepting of life.

Alcoholics Anonymous and 12-step programs in general encourage their participants to let go of unhealthy mind states and habits that were either precursors to addiction or that were entwined with the addict's life when she or he was "out there" using. The following list of letting-go possibilities is based on my own experience of working with both helpers and clients:

Pain and stories that support suffering

Criticism and judgment

Shame/self-hatred

Attempts at controlling people

Self-absorption

Tendency to deprive/harm oneself

Attachment to outcome

Insistence that reality conforms to fantasy

Impatience

Anger

Images about how you need to be

Entangled relationships

Self-righteousness

Being special

Comparing self to others

Focus on personal appearance

Drive for material acquisition

Sarcasm

Denial

Blaming others
Unexpressed grief

Resentment
Thinking you always know best
Striving for approval
Sense of separateness
Guilt

Having self-improvement efforts be
  opportunities for punishing self
Worrying
Filling time with intoxicants (drugs/
  computer/TV/sex)
Image of how children turn out
Thinking there is always an answer
Avoiding challenges
Rejection of the present moment
Fear

In general, letting go liberates us from: (a) our difficult past experiences and seemingly unmanageable lives; (b) our stuck and sometimes distorted (or in the 12-step tradition—"stinking") thinking involving personal judgments and shame; (c) rigid emotional states like despair, resentment, or anger; and (d) patterns of behavior or relationships that are not healthy or fulfilling. When *we*, as practitioners, let go of some of our own unhealthy baggage, we create more space to hold the struggles and pain of our clients.

In Zen, the out-breath equates with our letting go. We release the world that we had just inhaled, and we send it out to the universe without a clear sense of what the universe will do with it. We trust that the universe or God is big enough to hold our out-breath and, by implication, everything else that we release or let go of. This metaphor offers many important lessons for helping practitioners.

Because helping practitioners are human, we suffer from the same kinds of issues as everyone else. However, there are particular forms of thinking/feeling that arise in the helping process that are important to emphasize. In the middle of our interactions with clients, we slow down and engage in mindful breathing so that we develop the capacity to stop and identify patterns that emerge. We are less reactive and less controlled by strong feelings, habit, or unconscious thought processes. We see that the things we do, the way we feel, the responses we make, and the attitudes we have are not inevitable. They arise because of beginning-less causes and conditions, also called karma. We apply the intention of letting go in order to create shifts in karma, in other words to be less of a passive recipient of patterned or habitual behavior and feelings and to make a conscious effort to do everything we can to be an effective presence for the people whom we are helping. We examine *letting* go of the following elements seen as integral for helping practitioners: (a) attachment to outcome, (b) attempting to control people, (c) impatience and self-righteousness,

(d) sense of separateness, (e) fear, and (f) despair. We will see during these discussions that these elements are interrelated.

## Letting Go of Attachment to Outcome

There is a difference between working collaboratively with a client on her/his goal or aspiration and becoming attached to an outcome. Sometimes when we are attached, we are stuck in the mindset that things have to turn out the way we want them to. When our imagined results do not happen, we may blame ourselves or our clients, or become angry with our clients for not being better clients. We lose sight of how the helping experience is, in fact, a process that includes detours, uncertainty, failure, and reassignment of priorities. We also may become overly identified with results and take personally the absence of achieving particular outcomes.

At times, client situations that seem fraught with failure have positive consequences as they unfold. The client-worker journey may unfold in a manner that was not intended; however, outcomes may be advantageous in the long run. One time I worked with a woman who had struggled with disciplining her 10-year-old son John. Her initial goals involved becoming more effective in setting limits with her son. She also wanted to become more stable economically.

It soon became apparent that the mother had alcohol problems that made her day-to-day life chaotic and her day-to-day parenting unpredictable. Although she resisted entering treatment, she had been openly thankful regarding the opportunities that her son enjoyed when he would venture over to a neighbor's house and the couple would feed him and watch over him. The original parent-child focused goals that the mother and I had established shifted. Although, the situation at home was "good enough" and did not meet the threshold for a Child Protective Services report, the priorities in the case shifted to include working with the neighbors so as to assure and bolster their continued support in raising John. The intentions of all the parties were clear—they all wanted what was best for John. In a collaborative and non-blaming manner, the neighbors stepped up and said that they would be willing to adopt John and have John's mother visit him. John's mother made the heroic decision of consenting to this plan even though her financial situation would be more uncertain as a result. The initial outcomes or goals as outlined were not achieved and the early stages of the case suggested failure and stagnation. The eventual outcome, however, was more positive than anyone—including John's grandparents (John's mother's parents)—could have envisioned.

This is one story of what can happen when we are able to let go of outcomes. Other stories are not so positive. We let go of outcomes because we know that ultimately we cannot control what happens. We intend to do our best and sincerely contribute our efforts to the helping process.

## Letting Go of Attempting to Control People

Some of us enter this field partially possessing the delusion that we would be able to control people and get them to do what we think is in their best interest. We may have failed in these very same efforts with our family members; now we try our dirty work on our clients. As we embark on helping others, it is important that we let go of our tendencies and inclinations to control people. We find that in a particular case we are distressed because a client is not as motivated as we think he should be or because he continues to engage in problematic and self-destructive behavior. The source of our confrontations with clients is not the detached stance of the practitioner who allows the client to have his or her own life; instead, it is of the practitioner who is angry and frustrated that the client is not engaging the way that the practitioner believes that he or she should.

Our breath helps us return to a strong back, soft front state of detachment. This state is not characterized by noncaring nor by dull and spacey apathy. Detachment embodies love of the client as well as the open-hearted acceptance that we cannot control the client's journey. (In fact, we really cannot even fully control our own journey.) We may still feel anger and disappointment regarding our clients' seemingly stupid decisions and self-sabotaging behavior; however, we are able to let go of these emotions and judgments and not have them define the way we feel about and act with our clients.

## Letting Go of Impatience and Self-Righteousness

Being attached to outcomes or seeking to control leaves us vulnerable to becoming impatient. We begin to realize that others are not conforming to our plan, not behaving as we think that they should, and are not seeing the world as we do, and soon we can hardly stand listening to them and their nonsensical ways. In my experience, these kinds of dynamics occur not only in terms of practitioners and clients but relatively more often among colleagues, between supervisors and supervisees, and among students in professional preparation programs. It seems that for many of us, clients may get more of our open-hearted, radically accepting nature. We commit ourselves toward being nonjudgmental with them and we, perhaps, sense that their problems and struggles give them permission to have funky attitudes or unpredictable behavior. People whom we consider to be peers—such as agency colleagues and fellow students—should be more like us. When *their* behavior is questionable, we have little tolerance or patience for it.

With clients, we make the determination to let go of our inclinations to become impatient and seek to understand the reasons that people act, think, and feel the ways that they do. The level of understanding that we apply for clients is, at times, not available for peers. Our thoughts and words are pointed while evaluating agency colleagues and student peers as too uncaring, too quiet, too immature, too racist, too homophobic, too needy, too authoritarian, too lazy, too angry, too inclined to throw race in your face, too narcissistic, too religious, too nonspiritual, too prone to counter-transference, too unaware, too irresponsible, or too emotionally fragile.

In these instances, we need to mindfully witness our reactions for what they are—impermanent judgments and feeling states. We do not have to get stuck in them and, thus, we decide to let them go. We can begin with a fresh slate regarding our colleagues, supervisors, and supervisees. We release our stories about who the other is and we begin anew. We notice that differences start to make us uncomfortable and we apply compassionate awareness to the source of the discomfort. We look at our discomfort and arising impatience with a degree of equanimity and steady breath. We let go of our righteousness and impatience and we open our hearts, radically accepting the person in front of us.

## Letting Go of Separateness

Our clients' and colleagues' journeys are entwined in our own. Sometimes in reaction to our sense of powerlessness, we distance ourselves from our clients and begin to use labels or engage in what one supervisee referred to as "gallows humor." This kind of humor has the short-term gain of entertaining us in the face of an environment of pain and uncertainty. We take a vacation from the client's difficult and painful reality and enter a mindset that may be a slippery slope toward sarcasm, cynicism, and reinforcing the notion of "us and them."

Our sarcasm may be particularly destructive. Many times sarcasm involves an intention—however conscious or unconscious—to hurt or offend. Sarcastic language hides our own intentions even from ourselves and the derisive humor may appear innocuous. At times, sarcasm may be the first step toward greater separation from our clients and may enhance an individual mindset or agency culture of alienation.

We are wired for a fight-or-flight reaction toward situations that are perceived as dangerous, and we may perceive our clients' pain or struggles as threatening to our well-being. A reflexive, organic response in the face of threat is to compartmentalize the struggles as belonging to the other; derisive humor as well as the over-intellectualization of client problems assists us in this process. As we cultivate this kind of mentality while working with clients, we become less inclined to truly touch their pain and, in fact, may become numb to who they are or to what they are actually dealing with. As this process progresses over time, we become less inclined to open to the real-life world of the client and become less believing of his or her capacity for change. Not wanting to feel sadness, grief, and disappointment becomes our norm for engagement.

The core theme of this distancing process is separation. Through labels, insensitive humor, and eventually uncaring behavior, we reinforce to ourselves that we are on separate paths that are not interconnected. The client's path is fraught with troubles and difficulties and the practitioner's path increasingly becomes maintaining a professional distance and taking cover.

Our task is to let go of our sense of separation from our clients. We let go of our inclinations to protect ourselves with sarcasm and gallows humor, and we incline our minds toward our common fate. We allow ourselves to maintain healthy boundaries, but we tune into how our lives are ultimately tied together. We let go of our fear and embrace the contradiction of boundaries and oneness.

## Letting Go of Fear

The process of letting go—regardless of the issue—tests the degree to which we can address our fear. Fear is the primary reason that we are holding on in the first place and the reason that we are holding on so tightly. We are afraid to change our patterns of doing things, afraid of incorporating new ideas, afraid of opening our hearts to pain, and afraid to radically accept people and situations. Some students report that they are afraid to embody a soft front because they feel vulnerable, and others report that they are afraid to embody a strong back because it does not coincide with the kind, benevolent image they have of themselves.

When we apply compassionate awareness or mindfulness, we look at our fear and are not afraid of it. As Thich Nhat Hanh has said, "We invite fear into the house for a cup of tea but we do not offer it anything else." Fear will visit occasionally; sometimes it has something useful to say, and eventually it will leave. We do not have to exert effort to make fear comfortable while it is having tea with us, and we do not have to indulge it. We also are advised not to suppress it or push it away. Fear, like other feeling states and thoughts, grows nastier and more intrusive when we attempt to suppress it or stuff it into a closet.

Sometimes, our manner for letting go of fear is simply to witness its presence while we go about doing our activity. Many times when I introduce an exercise in class or in a supervision group, I am aware of fear arising within me. I notice the adrenaline shooting through my body, and I mindfully breathe. I do not engage in a war between my calm slow breath and my fast-beating, fearful heart. I let fear have its place and let it lose its grip over time. As we see in the last chapter, we encounter fear when shedding our armor and when swimming upstream against convention. We apply the intention of letting go of fear. We release it into the universe (or if it makes sense to you, we give it to God). We give ourselves and our clients a gift when we let go of fear. Our intimate experience of letting go allows us to mentor our clients in letting go of their own fears of engagement and change.

The discussion of fear as a force flowing through us is comparable to a narrative approach to emotional states. Fear is universal. It has an essence that is experienced in organisms throughout the world. As we tune into this reality, we see that naming fear strictly as "mine" is like naming oxygen as my oxygen. Fear is a river that will at times run through us. As we witness it, breathe through it, not feed or indulge it, we become successful in our intention to let it pass through us.

## Letting Go of Despair

Despair seems available to many of us. Maybe a crisis sets the conditions for despair to arrive. Other times small acts or critical words open the door, or perhaps it is our clients' pain or their difficulties that send us down this path. Despair is sometimes the cynical disguise of grief. As you breathe, you consider whether it makes sense to just feel sad about the struggles and difficulties around you. You experience these feelings and then you commit to engaging in activities or contemplations that create joy. Again, we navigate that delicate balance between pushing away despair and going through the process of accepting the feeling, seeing if it is linked to an emotion such as grief or sadness, experiencing the feeling, and replacing it with an emotional state that is beneficial for ourselves and our clients. Our overarching intention is to let go of despair because we benefit our clients when we are optimistic and can project joy. We owe it to our clients to let go of despair because our client's fate is somewhat connected to our own, and they will "catch" our negative worldview or depressive nature if we are particularly stuck.

## MINDFULLY EATING RAISINS

Jon Kabat-Zinn (1990) utilizes mindfulness exercises with clients in his ground-breaking stress reduction work at Massachusetts General Hospital in Boston. Zen student and psychologist Marsha Linehan (2003) involves her emotionally volatile and sometimes suicidal clients in similar exercises. One exercise that can be practiced at home or collectively in a classroom is eating a raisin. Students reported at semester's end that the collective experiencing of the following simple exercise was profound:

- Whether this exercise is done individually or in a group, create the intention that the environment is to be quiet.
- Allow yourself (yourselves) to be grounded in your breath.
- Take one raisin in your fingers and notice the raisin's appearance and texture.
- Put the raisin in your mouth and mindfully chew it. Notice thoughts and feelings that arise and come back to the activity of eating the raisin.
- Take your time. Let yourself taste the raisin and feel the raisin moving through your mouth. Chew the raisin at least 10 times.
- When you are ready, swallow the raisin and return to your breath.
- Reflect on and discuss what happened for you during this exercise.

Eating a raisin can be a powerful and memorable metaphor that illustrates possibilities for mindful practice. We can eat the raisin and barely be aware that we are eating a raisin. We can eat the raisin and be aware of many passing thoughts, feelings, and judgments about the exercise, and then come back to the raisin. We can be quite present for the activity of eating the raisin. All alternatives present lessons and the raising-eating experience will be different for us each time.

## CULTIVATING POSITIVE STATES

We live in a society where the government often tries to frighten us and the media overstimulates us. Images of violence, scandal, and falls from grace are common. In addition, many of us have suffered from violent acts or difficult experiences. We may feel inadequate, oppressed, and cynical. Despite our difficulties, clients need us to shine light on a path that seems worthy to pursue. To some degree, we as practitioners become that light and the model of a life worth living.

The degree to which we project joy and the sense that life is beautiful is immensely important. I consistently see clients appreciate their helper's positive outlook and smile; on the other hand, I have witnessed clients who do not gravitate to practitioners who project a dismal worldview or personal despair.

How much we incorporate a mindful approach to our life affects the degree to which our life will be balanced. When I am not mindful and sink onto the couch for 6 hours of football viewing, I emerge from the experience irritable and unfulfilled. When I am mindful about what is healthy for me, I generally watch 1 or 2 hours of football (I am not a saint) and do other things—like walking or spending time talking to my family members—that bring balance and joy into my life. Although we are often not aware of it, we are faced with these kinds of choices all the time. We can live our lives on automatic pilot, barely aware of what we are doing and how we are living moment-to-moment, or we can tune into the present moment and make decisions about what is healthy for us. Thich Nhat Hanh points out that these decisions—which appear to be private—actually affect the well-being of the entire world.

Think about how we listen to the radio as we drive in our car. At certain intervals, commercials are broadcast. The volume increases and we are assaulted with exaggerated claims designed to get us to buy things. The sounds are intrusive; they are engineered to be memorable and sometimes the strategy for being memorable means that the advertisements are calculated to be obnoxious. Our primary activity when driving a car is driving a car. If we have turned the radio on, our secondary activity is listening to music (or perhaps talk radio). We often approach the activity of driving and listening to the radio—just as we do many things in our lives—in a nonmindful way. One, two, three, four, five, six commercials in a row come blaring into our car as we drive toward our destination. Our comatose nature is the only reason we would tolerate such an assault on our senses. Do we have the courage to wake up, do things differently, and turn off the radio?

In Zen, mindful activity is a profound act. In the grand scheme of things, whether radio commercials are penetrating your particular mind seems to be quite insignificant. The Zen approach is that our activity directed toward cultivating positive mind states creates a ripple effect benefiting the universe. It is the drop in the ocean that Mother Teresa said would be missed were it not there. Thus, the application of practitioner mindfulness extends beyond the immediate client-practitioner encounter. We take care of and protect our minds as well as cultivate joy and happiness in our lives in order to be present and helpful for our clients. This kind of attention is the antidote to personal burn-out and compassion fatigue. We check in with ourselves and our environments and find the discipline to pursue health and balance. Many times the healthy choices involve seeking the support of others, other times it may involve taking care of our bodies, doing things that feel creative or fulfilling, listening to music, engaging in a spiritual practice, breathing mindfully, or resting.

## MINDFULNESS AND SOCIAL RESPONSIBILITY

We engage in mindfulness as we are in space with others. We bring an intention to contribute positively to the well-being of the group and with other individuals in our presence.

A recent class experience brought home the need to emphasize that mindfulness is not a solitary activity—that is, me and my mindfulness. Although students in class had opportunities to reflect on how they were becoming more present and mindful with their clients, when they engaged in small-group activities with peers, they were sometimes unfocused, not so respectful, judgmental, and dismissive. As with many classroom experiences, there was a range of commitment levels regarding their constructive involvement with the exercise, attention to the growth of fellow group members, and consistency in being present.

We had a classroom discussion regarding the importance of applying mindfulness to our intentions and our interactions with others. What is our intention when we hear that we have a group exercise to accomplish? Do we go through the motions, fight with the exercise, and protect ourselves? Or do we bring our focus on making a positive contribution, attending to the needs and experience of others, and navigating through our own barriers toward full participation?

We mindfully move our chairs to form our small groups and tune into our intentions as we prepare to sit down together. We bring our concentration to the task at hand and contemplate the following questions:

- What role will I play in this exercise?
- How will I serve the group through my communication?
- How will I attend to group members who are more reluctant to talk?
- What will I do with the judgments that arise as I interact with others who have ideas and communication styles different from my own?

Classroom and small group experiences are framed as opportunities to practice mindfulness. We do not just eat a raisin and see what kinds of effects the experience has on our helping practice. *Mindfulness is integrated into our lives and all of our interactions become the ground for its application.* In the classroom, we have the chance to do things as we normally do—somewhat self-absorbed and wired for self-preservation with an eye on the professor's perception of our performance. We also have the opportunity for thoughtful and committed participation, grounded in our steady breath. Within this commitment, we attend to the interconnected nature of our work as a class and we get in touch with our capacity to help others. Although often depicted otherwise, the journey in the classroom is not a solitary one in which each individual—with varying degrees of effort—strives to get an A.

The class did respond to this discussion. Group discussions became more respectful and contained fewer disruptions. I observed instances where members took it upon themselves to create space and draw out more reluctant participants.

This is the same kind of discussion that we need to have with our clients as well. We seek their mindful participation in group, not because this kind of involvement makes them "good clients" who are pleasing us as practitioners, but because their focused participation sets them on a path of freedom. As clients connect with each other, their internal selves, and their moment-to-moment experience, they taste what it is like to truly live one day at a time. Practitioners are able to have these kinds of conversations with clients when we ourselves are living this kind of life.

## FORGETFULNESS

Forgetfulness may be the biggest barrier to mindful practice. When a student approaches me before class, I am half-heartedly with her during our conversation. I am concerned about the sequencing of my PowerPoint slides and a short clip from the Internet that I will show to the class. What will I do first? How much delay will there be as I transition back and forth from the slides to the clip and back to the slides? Having the laptop as a major accessory in the class still makes me uncomfortable, and I start thinking about whether I could or should try to integrate all this technological stuff. Oh yes, there is a student who is speaking with me.

I forgot to mindfully tune into this student's presence as she stood before me. I could have either dropped the laptop stuff for a few minutes and really have listened to her (which I often do) or I could have told her that I wanted to give her the attention that she deserved at another time—such as during the break or after class. Instead, I missed what the moment was truly about and I divided my attention between the laptop and the student. Because I am not comfortable with technology and because I am a stickler for starting class on time, the student received less and less of my attention until the point came when I hardly knew what she was talking about or why she was standing in front of me.

Habit energy related to being distracted and acting hurried took over. I had forgotten what a precious opportunity it was to mindfully connect with this wonderful student and allowed my mind to wander in various directions. This kind of sequence is repeated countless times in our lives, and many of our clients probably have received more than their share of this kind of treatment. Fortunately, my period of forgetfulness was shorter than it had been on other occasions. I woke up in an instant, when I saw the student walk back to her seat. I could sense the unsatisfactory quality of what had occurred between us and I stopped. I let go of needing to have everything in place with my laptop, and I addressed the overlooked student:

> Here I am talking about mindfulness and mindful interactions with clients. I am so focused on setting up for the class that I barely see who you are. I'm sorry about that.

We always have opportunities to come back to what is important. Sometimes, it is healing for ourselves and others to acknowledge that we have been away and to apologize. This gesture can be quite affirming for people who have customarily received only parts of people's attention and who perpetually feel confused about what they can expect from helpers or intimate friends or partners. In some client situations, punctuating our temporary absence with a declaration may compound the hurt. It may make more sense to note our lack of presence to ourselves, then reconnect without any fanfare. We live in forgetfulness rather than mindfulness a good deal of the time. We are moving fast, multitasking, and receiving countless messages regarding our inadequacy and the possibilities of greater happiness or fulfillment offered through the consumption of food, pharmaceuticals, alcohol, or products.

In terms of clients, we may forget and come to believe that a story about who they are—in the form of a diagnosis or problem statement—is in fact them. We also may respond in a fight-or-flight manner to their struggles (to be discussed further in Chapter 5). Just as we bring ourselves back to our breath, we bring ourselves back to the memory that our clients deserve our moment-to-moment presence and mindful attention. We let go of our forgetful haze, and radically accept ourselves for visiting the land of forgetfulness. We compassionately welcome ourselves back to the present moment and to the client who is sitting just a few feet away.

# Chapter Five

# CURIOSITY, COMPASSIONATE CARING, AND INSPIRATION

*Beyond Professional Warmth*

The chapters on strong back/soft front, radical acceptance, and mindfulness emphasized the practitioner's embodiment of spiritual, emotional, and mental states and ways of being while working with clients. In this chapter, we discuss more precisely the ways we learn and the actions we take with our clients. If we want to understand and act with and on behalf of the person sitting in the room with us, we need to commit to various levels of inquiry and ways of caring vis-à-vis this individual. In terms of learning about the client, the worker's journey is not as a sanitized scientist coolly "assessing" the other. This chapter advances an attitude or way of being that characterizes the way we learn from and about clients. Once again, because social work, counseling, and psychology texts present practitioners as emotionally and spiritually neutered individuals, a discussion of practitioner curiosity, caring, and inspiration rarely occurs. These elements are presented here, however, as essential to our strong back/soft front work.

## CURIOSITY

The curious practitioner approaches her or his client with the perspective: Please teach me about your life and about who you are—I will learn from you. The full implication of "teach me" refers to the practitioner's dropping preconceived notions of the client that are based on characteristics such as race, mental health diagnosis, foster care status, and so on. Practitioner stories emerge from our weaving together stereotypes based on client characteristics, diagnosis, and client history and facilitate our insertion of time-honored knowledge into interactions with our clients. As we act more and more from this so-called knowledge base, we may, in fact, get in our own way of truly understanding our clients and we may disempower the client from being an expert of her or his own story. As I wrote some years ago:

> Knowledge—rather than engagement in deep listening with a calm, receptive mind—can lead a worker to enter relationships with lenses that facilitate attaching meanings, categories, and labels based on the worker's (mind) rather than the client's experience. (Bein, 2003, p. 138)

At the time, I discussed the benefits of an ethnographic approach to practice that created an open field for the client and created the ground for us to drop our judgments, projections, and preformed stories. The ethnographic worker was to work inductively from the client's narrative and build understanding in that manner. Missing from this discussion, however, was the spirit of curiosity that I have come to see as vital to the helping endeavor.

Curiosity points to the practitioner's affective state when he or she is making contact and trying to understand the client's life. Embedded in our curiosity is our deep sense that learning about this individual is not about mechanically asking questions from an intake form nor is it related to solidifying or validating our quickly formed hypothesis about the client's struggles. Curiosity guides our questions and emerges from our intention of forming human connections with our clients. Some of our questions may help us or our clients to identify strengths, some of the questions may be useful to understand dynamics related to the problem at hand or to generate possible solutions, and some of the questions may relate to generating laughter, a sense of connection, or a sense that we are invested in learning about the client's life. When we are sincerely curious about the individual who sits before us, the line of questioning may not necessarily follow a linear progression related to historical facts or increasing dysfunctional behavior. The genuinely curious practitioner is willing to tolerate ambiguity and is willing to allow the client to weave his or her story amidst a backdrop of practitioner delight in learning who this person is.

In addition to delight, curiosity comes with an energy that transcends what the dispassionate scientist may bring to the encounter. We want to learn about the client's life because we *care* about her as well as wish to provide her help. The curious practitioner is not only listening to facts, but is listening to the nuances of the story and observing the client's affect. Our curiosity reveals our personal interest in the client's life, thus enhancing the client-practitioner connection in the midst of the telling. The curious practitioner is always open to additional possibilities.

When a special needs teenager complained about what he referred to as his parents' "useless advice," I wondered aloud with him what it would be like to start listening to his own advice. To what degree was he, at this point, prepared to decide what his day would look like if he were not to have so much energy directed at his parents' incompetence? My curiosity of these matters guided the inquiry. I did not, in fact, have a ready-made answer to these questions, nor did I have a sense of how he or his parents should proceed. Curiosity was the engine that fueled mutual exploration and discovery. Maintaining a posture of not knowing and being genuinely curious helped establish a radically accepting container as well.

Curiosity may also accompany an adventurous spirit that can pay dividends, both in terms of learning about your clients and in creating transformative opportunities. Recently, I read a poem that I thought could engage a treatment group whose clients were labeled as dual diagnosis. The spiritual poem, written by the Persian poet Hafiz (see Ladinsky, 1999), offered images—the sun and the moon—that, I reasoned, they could access throughout the day and night. I believed that there were many useful metaphors in the poem and thought the poem could appeal to people with more or less formal beliefs regarding a higher power. I am constantly curious about substance abuse clients' actual understanding and implementation of the spiritual aspects of the 12 steps. Additionally, I have been curious regarding our program's ability to engage on a group level with our clients regarding how they make sense of the role of spirituality in their recovery.

My curiosity about the group's response to the poem was not so much a scientist's curiosity, but more a curiosity regarding how I could make a difference with the participants. It was the first meeting of January: would metaphorically tying this poem to the New Year help people engage or see the relevance of its content? Would the unique and fresh demand that the clients relate their interpretation of art to their spiritual practices, or my willingness to be vulnerable with a new activity make the group more worthwhile than the usual group format? Clearly, the energy was higher in the group than at other moments. One participant in particular who struggled with the concept of God seemed particularly invigorated. At the very least, there was a format for everyone to discuss their particular spiritual practices—whether they related to the poem or not. As the group session progressed, some members felt increasingly thankful that this new challenge was presented to them. One member was angered about the use of metaphors—sun and moon—when the straightforward idea of God should be all anyone would need. The diversity of expression and client need was a delightful result; the curious person welcomes this kind of diversity (including beliefs about the weaknesses of the practitioner's efforts).

Curiosity about clients does not always proceed in a nonlinear fashion nor does it necessarily involve creative issues like poetry. Sometimes our curiosity moves along in such a manner that we collect information related to social or psychological dynamics, behavioral patterns, or client or family history. In these instances, we allow for our knowledge to enhance our understanding of a client's situations. We, however, remain mindful of the potential pitfalls related to seeking information in such a way as to affirm ourselves or our sense of fixed knowledge. As we construct our practitioner story about who the client is, what her diagnosis is, or what strengths she has, we may selectively listen and, thus, be attending more to our elegant mind and its projections than to the client herself.

Even embracing a strengths' orientation with clients makes one vulnerable to this pitfall. An individual may really want the practitioner to understand how life's conditions and the client's present emotional state have left her feeling devastated and in profound pain. If our ears are particularly attuned for client strengths while meeting with her, and we focus our efforts toward building a strengths' embedded narrative because "we know" how helpful it is to construct this story and feed it back to her, the client may experience that we are not understanding her. In fact, she may believe that we are minimizing her pain and she may have the ever-familiar sense that she is not being heard. Our knowledge about the strengths' perspective and its benefits, *in this case*, has led us down a path that is more a reflection of our ideological stance than about our tuning into the client's message or, perhaps, need. As we were building knowledge concerning the client's strengths, creating a scenario in our mind about how we would share our view of her strengths, then mentally tying it all up with notions about how helpful this would all be, we were traveling down the path of knowledge and theory that took us further and further away from our client with each step.

As we take our position with our strong back and soft front, we do not incline ourselves to the right or the left or, in other words, toward any ideological stance or emotionally charged state. We just show up and become present with the client. Our curiosity grows from the ground of love rather than from our predisposition to find out just what is wrong or to prove correct our elegant ideas or prewritten stories about the client's life. Similarly, our strong upright back allows us to sit in the middle of client and worker pain and uncertainty, and our healthy curiosity emerges from this stable and expansive posture. When our backs are weak or our posture slumped or leaning in one direction or another, it is as if—as Zen teacher Ed Brown described during a retreat—we are either ducking from the possible difficulties that the client may throw our way or leaning into our particular, familiar pattern of response that is more about us as practitioners than about our clients' needs.

A strong back alone, however, can create rigidity and difficulty with processing unexpected information. Strong back curiosity can also create practitioner-client conditions similar to a mechanical intake interaction, where the practitioner fires away with the questions on the form, listening just enough to record responses and, perhaps, an occasional "I'm sorry that happened." However, it is the soft front that allows the practitioner to be moved by the client's story and who the client is. From this soft front, the worker sets the course of further exploration on a road that is filled with the practitioner's compassion. In the middle of my questions with a recent client, I let myself be touched by her hurts, her challenges, her triumphs, her resilience, and her courage to persevere. There was no separation between my curious self and my deep admiration of my clients' courage. As our time was ending, I reflected on her courage to deal so beautifully with her own brain injury, family alcoholism, abuse, parental schizophrenia, and limited financial and personal support. My comments to her at the end of the session flowed from a body-mind experience of venturing with her through the telling of her life's story as well as my sense of being honored through spending an hour with this wonderful human being. At the end of the session, my words, "You are a courageous woman," emerged from a heart of love and compassion.

The lotus often serves as a metaphor in Buddhism and is quite useful here. The lotus makes its home in the mud or the swamp, and often when we are with clients, our task is to sit with them in this swamp of their struggles, pain, challenges, despair, grief, fear, and difficulties. As we hang out in the swamp of our clients'—and ultimately our own—lives, we become rooted in the ways of the swamp; we develop facility in sitting with dignity amidst suffering and are able to be nourished in the environment. The open lotus displays the flower or heart that brings compassion and presence to even the most difficult circumstances. We are that lotus flower, and as we sit with our clients, we teach them to be that flower as well. We, as does the lotus, ask for nothing in return and we require little to be this kind of presence for our clients. Our ability to maintain equanimity and solidity establishes the ground for sincere, open-hearted curiosity and acceptance. The following example discusses the value of a nondefended self as an element of equanimity.

## Curiosity and a Nondefended Self

Recently, Tom, a group client, was fidgeting and he appeared to be disgusted in the middle of the group's session. When I called on him to check in, he stated that he wanted to pass because he was doing fine and he wanted to let other group members—who were more in need than he was—have his time. After all, Tom said, the group process was breaking down and some people were laboring on unnecessarily about problems that could have been more quickly wrapped up. Without saying so directly, he implied that as a result of my lack of leadership with slower group members and my unfairness that led to an uneven distribution of time for group members, various people were getting the short end of the stick. Tom wanted to rectify the situation by passing on his turn to speak.

As Tom was talking, I tuned into my posture, sat up fairly straight, and breathed. My heart opened, and the feeling from the arrow that I thought he had slung my way barely registered. Instead of lapsing into defensiveness or small-mindedness, I wanted to know what all this meant for Tom. What does fairness mean for him? Would he be able to tolerate attention even in the face of his request to pass? Would he be able to hear my perspective and the perspectives of other group members concerning the issue of time? How would he feel about engaging in the group now that he had the opportunity to voice a frustration and complaint? Would he be able to nondefensively consider a connection I would make between what was happening with him in group and the progress he was making in his recovery? These questions emerged from a heartfelt sense of curiosity that I had about Tom, this group, and his path to either recovery or jail.

Tom believed that each group member should have an even amount of time, and his sense of fairness was further in evidence when, later on during his check-in, he insisted I call on a member who, he noticed, had raised her hand before he did. I complimented Tom on his willingness to let the group and me know what was going on and for being willing to air his complaint. My energy had to be dedicated to maintaining open-hearted curiosity regarding what would be beneficial for Tom as well as dedicated to turning this interaction into an opportunity for increased intimacy. It seemed that the possible consequences from Tom's risk could have been Tom feeling heard and increasingly connected or Tom feeling frustrated. If Tom had experienced significant frustration, Tom and I (and perhaps Tom and the group) could have been alienated from one another.

I asked about Tom's perspectives and desires regarding time allotment. He stated that he thought everyone should have the same amount of time to check in. I respectfully pushed forward, even though he had requested to pass because, I said, his contribution was too important to pass on. There was an excellent group discussion with varied opinions. Some discussion focused on how to decide which group member should go first during the process group. The other major topic involved whether equal time limits should be enforced, or whether it was important to be flexible about time allocations. Throughout the discussion, I made sure Tom was digesting the various perspectives. I believed it was also important for Tom to see that I consistently thought about the time. I rarely get caught up in trying to establish my credibility with clients; however, in this instance, I wanted Tom to know that my range of awareness included time allocation issues, apparent client needs on that day, whether all clients are in essence "working" or benefiting while one client is more thoroughly and deliberately sorting out particular dynamics, and the benefits that derive from the group's deep engagement in providing support, suggestions, and help. One thriving client stated, "We are all family here . . . people should get the time they need."

I wanted to know what Tom thought about the discussion, and he indicated that he could now see that there were other considerations regarding check-ins. Although we are not supposed to be self-disclosing at this setting, I told Tom that I often have sentiments in various settings that if I were in charge I would do things better then the appointed leaders. I wondered aloud if he had had these thoughts and felt that I could be truly accepting of whatever his answer may have been. I asked him to consider, however, whether this sentiment—which I equated with not surrendering—also *perhaps* hampered his recovery. Although I was deeply curious regarding his response to this question, I decided that because he requested initially to pass, I would ask him to sit with this question and we would discuss it during the next process group.

In the midst of Tom's frustration, he was faced with a fight-or-flight dilemma that, according to his history, appears to have been played out often. (I did not know about his history at the time this group incident unfolded.) In this instance, he expressed disgust and frustration (fight), and he wanted to pass and just be left alone after he dumped out his complaint (flight). Though I would not have been able to articulate this dynamic at the time, I maintained radical acceptance of the moment and curiosity about his reaction and how best to help. In the midst of this relatively minor turmoil, I faced Tom and his multiple reactions and thereby helped Tom face himself, the group, and me. I was not defensive regarding his criticism and believe that I, therefore, conveyed to Tom that his emotional life could be contained in the group.

Maintaining curiosity and an open-hearted or nondefended self creates space for clients to be their authentic selves. When the practitioner is nondefended, he or she helps to create a field where people sense that they do not have to dedicate energy to find out the right things to say in order to please the practitioner. Also, being nondefended projects to clients that it is possible to radically accept one's own shortcomings, failures, and actions or personal characteristics that others find worthy of criticism.

When we are nondefended, we can sit in the middle of being exposed and realize that hiding is not beneficial. Even if we feel some fear, we become aware that the taste of liberation occurs through maintaining authenticity. If fear sends us into temporary hiding, we suddenly realize that the shell we occupy, the mask we wear, and the lies or deceit we perpetrate are taking us and our clients off the path that we need to be traveling.

In this group example, I had lied in the middle of my description regarding the order in which I chose the clients to check in. I mentioned that I chose the person who wrote the lowest number on the attendance sheet (indicating they are not feeling well) to check in first, then I worked in order up the ladder until the people checking in at the end of the group had written that they were a "10" for the day. As the discussion progressed, I told the group that I had lied. I, in fact, used the check-in numbers as only one input regarding the order of the check-ins. Some of the decision making regarding check-in order was intuitive—I told them that I smell all of them as they enter the room—it was based some on who had time the week before, and so on.

In a program that defines honesty as integral to health, it seemed important for me to demonstrate my commitment to honesty and to untangle any knots inside me that would arise from lying. While I was declaring to the group that I had lied, I noticed that I felt freer and enjoyed a sense of even greater connection with the group.

This small act emerged from and enhanced the soft front work that is so important. My deep sense of caring for both the group and my own integrity pushed me to reveal a part of my process that fear may have prevented me from sharing.

Caring for clients and self does not, however, lead us to be an open book for our clients. Traditional helping profession discussions regarding boundaries are important and have parallels to Buddhist guidelines involving *right speech*. It is important that we are honest; however, it is also important that our speech is beneficial. Saying things to clients that compromise their sense of safety or confidence in the process or that are hurtful—all in the name of being honest and open—may be more about practitioner self-indulgence or *carelessness* than about practitioner *caring*. Our caring for clients ultimately guides how we apply principles discussed throughout the book.

## CARING FOR OUR CLIENTS

How
Did the rose
Ever open its heart
And give to this world
All its
Beauty?
It felt the encouragement of light
Against its
Being,
Otherwise,
We all remain
Too
Frightened.

—Hafiz translated
by Daniel Ladinsky

Caring is the light against our being that opens our hearts to the stories, pain, and aspirations of our clients. We care about our clients and communities so we return time after time with strength in our spine and an open, soft heart. In the midst of our own life problems, conflicts or irritations with the service setting, or frustrations with the clients themselves, our caring keeps us connected, compassionate, and committed to help. If we did not care so, we would succumb to fears of our clients' or our own pain, and our help—as Hafiz's poem suggests—would lack open-heartedness and beauty.

The idea of caring barely registers in traditional social work, counseling, and psychology scholarship and training. In one well-written, comprehensive text considered a classic for teaching social work foundation practice, Lawrence Shulman did not choose to discuss the concept of caring. Near the place that caring would be in the text's index if it had been included, there are 17 subtopics related to *contracting* involving approximately 100 pages of the 884-page book, while another nearby index listing, *deviant group member*, encompassed 12 subtopics and 28 pages. Despite this omission, caring actually forms the foundation of our work in the helping fields. Countless times when I have asked people to identify ingredients of a helping relationship that they had defined as positive and beneficial, the first thing they say is that they thought that the professional helper cared about them.

Caring in our professional relationships establishes the basis for clients where they can experience and begin to believe in what John Welwood (1996) describes as one's "inner core goodness." People develop this sense within an environment where they are fully seen and where they have their inner core goodness reflected. Thus, in one of the few human service books that highlights the value of caring, Diana Rauner (2000) features *attentiveness* as its foundational component.

Professional caring can seem almost like a contradiction in terms. People from diverse ideological perspectives may argue that caring should reside in the family—a traditionally conservative view—or that the very mention of caring inherently devalues and feminizes the scientific legitimacy and professional preparation of a seriously trained cadre of social workers, counselors, psychologists, and medical providers—a traditionally liberal view. Rauner (2000) addresses what I am simplifying as the conservative view and asserts that professional caring is meant to complement, and not be competitive with, family caring. She suggests that, particularly with adolescents, human service caring can be integral to a community and bolster family caring and functioning.

The view more often represented in professional circles, labeled previously as liberal, so much emphasizes assessment of the other and intervention on behalf of the other that caring—which involves the inner life of the practitioner— escapes the dominant paradigm. (Within medicine, the terms *nursing care* or *medical care* are used; however, *care* in this context refers more to meeting needs directed toward health outcomes than anything having to do with practitioner intention or creating a field of compassion and validation.) Yet, it is caring that fuels our sincere intent to attend and to connect. The fact that we care about our clients helps us show up and act on their behalf even when we are irritated, tired, or in despair. Caring is the "encouragement of light" that opens our clients' hearts to worlds of possibilities and risk-taking and the increased sense that they are *worth* being cared for. Our clients naturally sniff for caring whether it is in the form of returned phone calls or e-mails, thoughtful and focused attention, or true intentions to benefit them and to act on their behalf. It is the pure, caring heart of the student intern that often means more to clients than the tried and true interventions of the seasoned professional.

We need to maintain deep awareness of the *degree* as well as the *skillfulness* of our caring and compassion during our work with clients. The degree to which we care for our clients will be influenced by our success in managing stress or distress in our lives or work site, our maintaining awareness regarding how present we are, our letting go of our frustrations and judgments with our clients, and our ability to dedicate and focus sufficient energy our clients' way. The skillfulness of our caring will be affected by the nature of our compassion directed toward our clients and how well we negotiate the dynamic of boundaries. The elements related to skillfulness of caring call for our strong back.

As mentioned, our acts of caring deeply resonate with our clients. When we care, we communicate an important message:

Yes, you are important. I am with you because I would like for you to be happy. You, your life, and how successful you will feel at the end of this process truly matter to me. The fact that being with you is part of my job only sets the ground for our interaction. If you need me to go beyond the usual limits of the job in order for you to receive benefit, I will do what I can to go the extra mile. Being with you is a sacred event; I will pay attention to you the best I know how. Please let me engage with you and please teach me about your life. Although I know some things about people who have had similar situations and struggles, I will do my best to not assume that I know and instead respect your sense of the way things are. Part of caring about you means I will give you space to express yourself, and I will not get defensive if you should have criticisms of me or this work site.

At times we will struggle with boundaries and rules. I will not be sure how much to bend agency rules or advocate for you, and how much to enforce agency rules and teach you how the structure and even, at times, the rigidity supports your success. At those times, you may think I am full of crap, and perhaps the most caring thing I will do in these instances is to hold my ground even in the face of your anger with me.

Sometimes while I am caring for you, I may become overly invested in the outcome to the point where I have put my own ego on the line. I will do my best to recognize these moments and to let go. I will say, "I'm sorry," when I make a mistake or when my actions hurt you. Sometimes, I may be lazy or tired and secretly hope that you do not show up at the office or that when I knock on your door you are gone. I will do my best on these days to be aware of my aversion and to find the energy and love to be with you in the way that you deserve.

I will risk being my authentic self, and I will do my best to keep your needs in the foreground. I will take care of myself so that my presence with you represents a time of healing and you can have the reasonable aspiration that working with me is better than working alone. I will do what I can to address your struggles or suffering, even engaging in actions that represent some kind of stretch, like advocacy on behalf of your needs or aspirations or confrontation, if I believe it will help you attain clarity and truth.

I will stay aware of the level of my caring. My intentions represent my emotional, attitudinal, and spiritual compass, and I vow to set them in the direction of caring for you.

## AWARENESS OF STRESS OR DISTRESS

Personal stress or distress weaving its way through our bodies and minds may compromise the soft front and strong back that we wish to offer our clients. As practitioners, we are not immune from difficult circumstances or painful feelings. When these kinds of situations or feeling states arise we need to witness them, be present for them, and find a way to enter our relationship with clients as open-hearted and solid as possible. When we are not consciously committed to addressing our difficulties, anxiety, or pain, we may act out our life troubles or inner emotional turmoil with our clients.

One part of this work involves giving yourself enough space to struggle in your life. As you are present with your own struggles, you open your heart toward yourself. As Stephen Levine puts it, you send love and compassion to yourself, rather than—what may be your custom—shame and hatred. You slow down and, perhaps, discover that quick fixes are not so much needed as holding yourself with compassion and forgiveness. Kim Phuc, famous as the Vietnamese girl running through her village with her arms burning from Napalm, now states that compassion and forgiveness are far more powerful than napalm bombs despite her lifelong suffering from burns resulting from the bombs' 1600-degree (F) heat. Ms. Phuc has since met, forgiven, and embraced one of the American military men who dropped bombs on her village that historic day. Her love and forgiveness has given him the strength to carry on after his post-Vietnam life had been largely broken. Ms. Phuc is able to forgive and openly embrace this U.S. soldier; *how much are you able to forgive and openly embrace yourself?*

We bring compassion for self, forgiveness of self, and presence into our interactions with others. Our open heart or soft front is not constricted, and the client experiences our sense of peace and caring. We are not deterred by the acts that our client has committed nor how demanding, scared, or angry he or she is. We create space for our client to grow, resolve difficulties, and feel supported and accepted.

Our open and caring selves may be compromised in the midst of challenges or low levels of personal awareness. High levels of stress or festering, unaddressed wounds may lean us toward approaching interactions with clients in a manner similar to our approach toward getting a haircut, something we need to accomplish in order to cross off an item on the day's to-do list. Our level of care is constricted, and clients—because they are so attuned to whether their practitioners care—become dissatisfied or alienated. Our words may be there in the form of advice, interventions, or feigned empathy; however, our clients know better.

## AWARENESS OF PRESENCE

Our quality of presence creates the caring environment that supports our clients. At times, our presence is deeply rooted in a foundation of radical acceptance and a strong back and soft front. Other times, especially if we are distracted or stressed, we may sell out our clients. In a clinical supervision session, a practitioner told me of his ambitious community work with a mentally ill client, about 35 years old, who had just lost her mother. This young woman was enormously dependent on her mother for food and shelter, companionship, and emotional support and sustenance. The practitioner actually did some wonderful work with the client regarding issues related to rent payment and financial matters; however, his approach lacked empathy for what she may have been going through. This woman was reportedly, before he arrived, curled up into a ball on the floor, and this practitioner did not see her beyond her financial needs. She was reduced, in fact, to these matters and in essence, part of her was invisible.

This supervisee is a beautiful, courageous, and insightful man, and he discussed how he is having so much difficulty managing stress from his job that he is running ragged most of the time. As he is doing so, he is missing some connections with clients and, perhaps, too often imposing solutions from his own perspective. Although he cares deeply for the well-being of his clients, his own stress level has compromised his soft front, and he has become overly focused on accomplishing tasks. His awareness of these dynamics is the first step toward realizing his sincere intention to skillfully care for his clients.

## CARING AND FOCUSED ENERGY

Sufficient energy is needed to actualize caring for and compassion toward clients. Compassion, according to Thich Nhat Hanh, involves our generous and resonating open heart as well as our willingness to *take action* to relieve pain and suffering. Compassion is the element of caring that spurs the professional helper to go the extra mile, to advocate, and to show up in the face of difficulty. If our energy is compromised or dispersed, we may fall short of our clients' needs despite our actual intentions or positive or even loving feelings for them. In the way we bring our mind to single-pointed attention in Zen, we must bring our mind-body into dedicated action on behalf of our clients.

Awareness of our energy level is essential for all human service providers. It is incumbent on us not to lapse into significant periods of *burnout* or *compassion fatigue* because of the suffering that ensues for our clients and ourselves when we are working under these conditions. Our compassion flows when our energy level is high, our outlook is positive, and our actions emerge from a base of mindfulness. We drive to a home visit with the radio off and we are aware of our deep, calm breathing. We nurture ourselves throughout the drive through our careful, focused attention, our nonaggressiveness, and our willingness to let go of a sea of swirling thoughts and stories. As we pull up to the home of our client, perhaps we are aware of a thought such as "maybe it would be better if the client were not there and I could just leave." We *stop* for a moment in front of the house and take care of ourselves and this thought. We breathe and feel compassion for ourselves and acceptance for the part of us that is inclined to flee because of fear or feeling sluggish. As we experience compassion for ourselves, we know that we must direct compassion and sufficient energy in the direction of our clients. We smile and begin to look forward toward making contact with the client. We have some idea about what we will speak about in the apartment that we are now in front of; however, we are beginning to embrace the reality that the primary ground of the visit that is about to occur is *not knowing*. We are willing to accept whatever fear we have about this uncertainty and we see the fear as a window into our client's experience and as an opportunity to be intimate with true fearlessness. We are prepared to be curious about this beautiful being's life and we begin to tune into the nonseparateness of our beating hearts. The seeds of this being and our own come from the same source; we were only watered in different ways. We allow ourselves to feel honored by the opportunity to be in the presence of this person. We know that we can hold and accept their emotions and their story. We have an opportunity to bring the gift of listening and caring and this individual is about to bring us gifts related to valuable teachings. When we enter the apartment and sit and face what is, we deeply connect to the truth. We also have the opportunity to let everything else—our ruminations about work, money, plans, family—drop away and we experience a sacred encounter. We knock on the client's door with a sense of deep joy and compassionate heart.

## CONTEMPLATION EXERCISE

What is your story as you begin to work with your clients? What needs to happen for you to be an energetic presence with your clients?

## Strong Back and Skillful Caring

One day a monk asked (Master) Chao-Chou to speak to him about Zen. Chao-Chou asked, "Have you finished your breakfast?" "Yes master, I have eaten my breakfast." "Then go and wash your bowl."
—Nhat Hanh (1995), p. 54

As we enter the apartment, our soft front greets our client. We sit on the client's couch and our strong back serves as the foundation for our emergent skillful caring. We begin our engagement with a sense of confidence about our journey. We accept whatever the client presents to us—anger, hope, reluctance, fear—and we listen to her story with deep caring and patience. The Zen metaphor is that we accept whatever is put in our begging bowl. Some days it is tasty, other days perhaps foul; some days it seems plentiful, other days barely a drop. We notice any reactions we may have toward what we receive; however, we do not cling to the reactions or get lost in them. We see them for what they are—temporary feeling states—and let them go.

"Go wash your bowl," cited above, refers to Zen's emphasis on practicality and simplicity. After we eat, we wash our bowl. We do not waste our time with such matters as dissecting Zen thought. We *wholeheartedly* do the next right thing, that is, washing the bowl. Additionally, washing our bowl is so mundane that no one will ever tell us what a great job we did. There is no ego gratification to be gained and whatever romantic or grandiose story we were telling ourselves about the special wisdom we were about to gain by being in the teacher's presence is put to rest.

When we fill out a consent form with the client, or we compliment her on a strength that we have just observed, we dedicate the same mindful attention to the activity as we would if we were to help her analyze major themes in her life. Zen is not about arranging hierarchies of activities on levels of importance. Washing the bowl in the monastery is not more or less important than discussing philosophy. Filling out a form or greeting a client is not more or less important than whatever else we may do in a session.

We eat from and wash our bowls in equanimity in the same manner that we take our seat and face the reality of our clients' and our lives coming together. We feel calm and confident knowing that the light of mindfulness is all we need. We become aware of our breath and this awareness becomes our anchor for the thoughts, feelings, and dynamics arising in the room. Grounded in our steady breath, we become deeply aware that we can hold whatever transpires. All we need to do is be intimate with what is; there is no reason to panic. If by chance, we do freak out over what is transpiring, we do not have to freak out about our freaking out. When we are able to meet our own fear or impatience with calmness, our frazzled state eventually recedes as does any emotional wave. In the midst of this calmness, we sense our interconnection and responsibility (i.e., ability to respond) with everything that happens in the room.

## Strong Back and Compassion

Compassion is the soft front response containing our aspiration to relieve another's or our own suffering. Our strong back establishes the structure for compassion and helps us engage in compassion that is skillful. Aura Glaser (2005) summarized elements of unskillful compassion or, as she put it, confusion about compassion. First, there is what Chogyam Trungpa called "idiot compassion." This kind of compassion *appears* to be kind, but may arise from the practitioner's intention to be liked or to avoid conflict. A genuinely compassionate act may, in fact, be sharp or pointed, and is not done for the ego gratification of being seen as nice or for receiving praise. True compassion respects the integrity of the client and fosters her empowerment. The truly compassionate act calls for us, at times, to take risks and engage in difficult encounters that clients may not necessarily appreciate.

A case example related to discharging clients at a substance abuse agency illustrates "idiot compassion." After hearing that two clients on his caseload would be discharged from the program, an agency practitioner was left with the task of informing his clients. Both clients had known that because of relapsing and/or infractions, they were in jeopardy of being discharged and during phone contacts each one asked the counselor about their status. In both instances, the counselor believed that the compassionate thing to do was to tell them over the phone that they were not to continue in the program. Why stretch the process out for them and make them come to the agency to hear the news? Why not spare them the trip to the agency, the extra embarrassment and public failure, and at least honor their wish to tell them their status during the phone conversation? As we explore this seemingly compassionate act, we find that sometimes it is more compassionate to have a meaningful—albeit more painful in the short-term—termination session than to say good-bye on the phone. This session would be an opportunity to face the truth of what is, even if it includes disappointment, anger, and fear. Facing reality without denial is exactly the lesson that we attempt to teach in the program.

Having the news come out at a face-to-face meeting and insisting that the client's status in the program could not be discussed on the phone would mean that the practitioner would have had to deal with not being nice and deal with the reality of the client's pain. Because this practitioner is courageous and dedicated to his own growth and client service, he could see that his so-called compassionate response may have been motivated by his wanting to be nice and accommodating, his own guilt regarding the clients' discharges, and his predisposition to avoid sessions that could be painful. In essence, his compassionate responses were not so compassionate.

A second form of unskillful compassion occurs when compassion is confused for attachment. While our attachments are volatile, sometimes conditional, and subject to whim, compassion is an inclusive field that we hold people in regardless of how they behave, how attractive they appear, or how they feel about us. We feel compassion for our client's pain whether we hear her story for the first time or for the fifth time. We commit to watching our feelings of irritation or devaluing thoughts wrapped in DSM labels arise, and we commit to letting them go and returning to our soft heart.

Finally, compassion may be unskillful when the practitioner's field is limited to *feeling* compassion and he or she excludes compassionate *action* on the client's behalf. Some practitioners equate the compassionate heart with being present for the client and listening. Compassionate action may involve stretching the boundaries of the agency or service setting and doing work that receives little notoriety. Our strong back can help us witness our own forces of inertia and our sense of helplessness as we navigate our way toward taking skillful action.

## CARING ACROSS DIVERSE POPULATIONS

Delusions are inexhaustible; I vow to transform them.
—Adapted by Joan Halifax Roshi
from Bodhisattva Vows

Caring and working across diverse ethnic/racial groups, sexual orientations, economic classes, levels of mental stability or physical wellness, genders, age groupings, and social strata poses challenges and opportunities. The practitioner can approach the reality of differences with a kind of naiveté sometimes found in Buddhist circles asserting how, essentially, we are all one. This view, however, is unworkable for helping practitioners.

Strong back wisdom involves our holding the reality that (1) people embrace the way in which they are different from others, that (2) there is a real social context involving people who sometimes mistrust and even dislike members of certain groups they consider as "others," and that (3) our minds are so deluded that we unknowingly believe that particular values and ways of thinking about the world are normative and universal.

The Zen approach is to embrace what is and fully enter it. Thus, we embrace the reality that the waters of diversity are choppy and unpredictable and the journey is full of unknowns. We engage with diverse clients with, perhaps, an even higher level of uncertainty than we do if some of our characteristics and tendencies more closely match. We are excited to learn about what situations mean to our clients, and we become acutely aware that our clients are there to teach us about their experiences as well as remind us that there are many points of view.

We perpetually let go of the belief that we "understand how things are" and we center ourselves on the ever-shifting ground. Zen practice teaches how to move with care and precision while engaging in various forms and rituals. The concentration attained from mindful and somewhat meticulous actions paradoxically sets the groundwork for personal authenticity and spontaneity. As we enter interactions with clients who are different from us—and of course, everyone is distinct on some level—we abide in a space that is dedicated to careful movement and protection of our clients, and we manifest spontaneity and risk-taking. This seeming duality, again, should be seen as two sides of the coin.

The part of ourselves dedicated to carefulness, nonharm, and having minimal impact emerges from recognizing the ways in which words can hurt as well as from understanding our clients' vulnerability to injury. Some people may have experienced traumas or years of mistreatment, difficulties, or abuse that has left them barely able to engage in meaningful dialog without feeling offended, attacked or, at the very least, invalidated. Our status and role as practitioners sometimes heightens the sense of vulnerability and sensitivity some clients already struggle with. As we sit with our clients, not only do we sometimes observe the divide between client and practitioner, we become aware that client fears and practitioner fears about differences are present in the room. We hold the fear and mistrust with care; we understand that in addition to the two of us in the room, there are historical misdeeds, social, family, and personal stories, and stereotypes. We tune into the degree to which a commitment to nonharm needs to guide our interactions. We cultivate the ability to act in this manner because there are times, such as when walking in nature, when we want to gently connect with the environment without damaging it. We pay attention to creating a container that feels safe and not too threatening. We may lean toward identifying and celebrating client strengths, and we focus on our wholehearted acceptance of the individual as she or he is.

We cannot only reside in carefulness, however. By *itself*, carefulness chokes off the kinds of opportunities for connection that demand genuineness, and without genuineness and spontaneity, the environment has a dead walking-on-eggshells feel. In the midst of our open-hearted willingness to take risks, we let our curiosity flow and we ask questions that some may consider taboo. We truly rejoice in the presence of the other and let ourselves be inspired and stimulated. We return to our breath and we cautiously contain our enthusiasm with a statement like: "Please tell me if that question was okay." Then we thank the client for how much we have learned through her or his risk-taking. In the spirit of practitioner risk-taking, we may share a perspective with a client and state how we recommend that she at least consider how this perspective has meaning for her life. The risk is that our words may offend the client, which has the potential to disturb the equilibrium established in the relationship and/or alienate the client from seeking further service. We tune into the part of ourselves that is hesitant to risk because of fears that the client may not like us or be upset with us. We function with the wider view that the way people feel about us is impermanent; it is constantly changing on some level.

We are mindful of our insecurity; however, we do not let our self-absorbed thoughts direct our approach. We decide whether to risk with clients based on our sense of what would be the most beneficial. Our relationship with a client may be stable and comfortable for us; however, there may not be much happening in terms of meaningful client transformation. We may need to push ourselves to move out of our comfort zone in order to have the client realize what is possible from the relationship.

Ironically, it is sometimes more of a risk for some practitioners to genuinely listen to their clients, attempt to understand their world, and maintain patience and balance while the client struggles. Some of us are more comfortable telling clients what to do, especially if there is a crisis or challenging situation at hand. In the midst of client difficulty or perhaps even physical danger, we may lean toward rigid responses that more reflect our fear or rush of adrenaline than our connection with the client and a clear understanding of the situation.

One case example brought up in clinical supervision is illustrative. A client who was 7 months pregnant reported in a group how she had been having consistent contractions that day and had other symptoms that perhaps indicated that she was beginning to go into labor. The practitioner reported that she was concerned about the client's cavalier attitude about the baby's status and the relative ambivalence the pregnant woman had as to whether she should seek medical care. Finally, the practitioner stated to the counselors and social workers in the supervision group that she thought that the client was being quite "self-centered" and she revealed how she lectured the client about the need to get to the hospital in order to take care of the baby.

My first response in the supervision group was to center myself. The way I can help practitioners stay connected with their clients is for me to stay connected with them. If I lecture practitioners about how they need to not lecture their clients, I will not be as effective. While centering myself, I came to a place of radical acceptance of the situation—the clinician's response—which I had judged as too nonempathic, and my hesitancy to say something different than the comments already made by the counselors and social workers in the supervision group. I first praised the practitioner for her concern about the baby's health and her willingness to be assertive. I also stated that given the constraints of the group structure—the place where the client revealed her situation—and the sense that the fate of the unborn baby's life was placed on the practitioner's lap, I may have done exactly the same thing as the practitioner if I had been the group leader in that situation. In other words, I attempted to establish a supportive and compassionate container through identifying the practitioner's strength, normalizing her response to the situation, and revealing that, perhaps it was only the benefit of hindsight that allowed me to offer an alternative to the way in which she worked with this client.

I pointed out to the practitioner that in the midst of her drive to make something happen and her simultaneously emerging judgments regarding the client's self-centeredness, she "was not with the client" during this time. I internally noticed that it was hard for me to deliver this statement to the supervisee, but I have come to understand that sometimes greater learning comes with clear correction; therefore, my intention has to be more aligned with practitioner learning and effectiveness than about being nice to them. This kind of intervention dilemma is also parallel to how practitioners themselves need to intervene with their clients.

I asked the practitioner and the supervision group members to imagine what may have been going on with his client that could have contributed to her struggle about whether she should go to the hospital. These kinds of speculations or hypotheses were designed to build a container of empathy so the client herself would not become invisible. Different agency counselors mentioned the possibility that because she had had two other children removed from her custody, the prospects of giving birth brought flashbacks of these traumatic incidents. One practitioner wondered whether she had at all bonded with the being inside her body. Another practitioner thought that perhaps she had recently used drugs and her appearance at the hospital would mean another colossal failure and the immediate removal of the newborn. If we as practitioners were at all touching the truth with our speculations, perhaps we were working with a client living with fear and a minimal connection with the baby. I suggested that as practitioners, we need to *be with the mother*—her fear, her sense of failure, her desire to flee or disappear or deny what was happening. We could still communicate urgency and, in fact, establish even clearer limits than the practitioner ended up establishing the night before. Rather than preaching and judging, our strong back, soft front intervention would have allowed us to deeply join with the client as well as define a structure for her to follow.

One practitioner whose wife recently gave birth to a premature infant confessed how he initially became inpatient with my softhearted approach with this client. He wanted to "make it happen"—that is, get her into the hospital. By the end of the discussion, however, he realized that being with the mother was more likely to produce a positive outcome, and that the mother's being seen and heard had ultimate value as well. In fact, he realized, taking a demanding posture with her about her need to save the being inside her body could easily reinforce the alienation and lack of bonding that the pregnant woman was experiencing.

Building knowledge through the practitioners' own recovery and social service experience helped the group change the story about the client being selfish and irresponsible and needing to be scolded about what to do. Instead, the story about the client included personal pain, fear, and confusion. The new story was about someone who needed both engagement with the client group and counselor and firm, caring structure about the next steps to take.

## Helpfulness of Knowledge about Diverse Populations

Knowledge about cultural or diverse population tendencies can be useful. In one situation that I was involved with, an elementary school teacher and principal were frustrated with a Hmong family's lack of follow-through with the school nurse's recommendation that an 11-year-old student be fitted for a hearing aid. Having knowledge regarding the Hmong community's lack of trust of Western medicine helped me be present for their aversion to the school, as well as present for the school's frustration and confusion regarding the family. If I had entered the situation with the Zen beginner's mind, a deluded view—that these parents were neglectful and uncaring—could have become my view. Another outcome of a beginner's mind could have led to my spinning around with the family and school in a swamp of mistrust and stereotypes. Cultural knowledge enhanced the strong back container that provided clarity as well as a structure where different perspectives could be held and heard. The family, in this situation, did eventually pursue medical options and coercion was not involved.

With one client, a number of years ago, my cross-cultural ignorance led to the client's discontinuing service with me. A Filipino man in his early twenties was seeing me and talking about his sense of feeling stuck in his life. He felt particularly responsible for the well-being of his large family who were residing back in the Philippines and frequently sent money to them despite the fact that he, himself, was struggling financially. I brilliantly applied the concept of co-dependence to his situation and suggested that he needed to focus on his own well-being before he could worry about his family's. Although he tried to tell me about the expectations placed on Filipino first sons, I "knew" that his explanations were a mere cover for unhealthy, co-dependent behavior. Once he learned about how co-dependent he was and he emerged from his denial, I envisioned positive gains. Even though he had seen me five or six times and our relationship was moving along nicely, he never showed up again.

Some may read this example and believe that they would not make such an obvious error. Buddhist practitioners, in particular, may think that they would be astute enough to identify judgments and let them go. I can only say in this regard, that because we live in a deluded world, we often do not understand how our judgments, areas of ignorance, and stereotypes operate. We also are sometimes oblivious to the manner in which we embrace our points of view and believe that they represent absolute truth. Any group of people—and Buddhist or Zen Buddhist groupings are no exception—can develop a sense of group-think that inevitably devalues the "others" and retains blind spots regarding diverse thoughts or experiences. Further, it is not uncommon for people who have not suffered with particular challenges to overlook or not connect with pain experienced by people who have different kinds of experiences or to minimize the mistrust that may arise when diverse people come together.

Ultimately, our approach is to acknowledge uncertainty for what it is. We enter complex interactions with a sincere, open heart. We care about our clients' and our colleagues' well-being and we recognize that our words are powerful. We tread with care and at the same time we are not too careful. Intimacy arises when we approach the other with our genuine selves and when we come to realize that, ultimately, there is one beating heart that brings us together. We hold the contradiction of oneness and diversity as we continue on our journey. We hold ourselves in compassion for the difficulties we will have, the connections we will experience, and the mistakes we will make.

## CLIENTS AS INSPIRATION

I remembered how it seemed like Barry would never meaningfully engage in the program. He loved to talk about his truck and flirt with a 22-year-old woman who was at least 30 years younger than he was. "Did you get a sponsor yet, Barry?" "No, well sort of, well there was one guy and he didn't really work out and I haven't had time to get another one," he would say. "How has your work been going on your steps?" we would ask him. "Well, I just can't seem to open the book to do them (literacy was not the issue). . . . I can't seem to do anything that I am supposed to do."

After about 2 months of running in quicksand, Barry gave himself and the rest of the group a taste of what it was like to be genuine. He admitted when he was questioned about his commitment that he had not been working sincerely at all and, he added, "My mind is still in such a fog that I can hardly move forward."

I remember being touched by Barry's honesty. His comments were not about trying to "get off the hook" or diverting the practitioners and the group members. His back, figuratively, was against the wall and somehow he felt safe, courageous, and/or desperate enough to tell the truth about how he was failing and about how lost he was. Time seemed to stop during that moment in the way that it does when clients inspire us.

Six months later, I experienced the same kind of sensations during Barry's advancement ceremony. The group members reflected on the ways in which Barry courageously peeled back calcified layers of protection and façade to "get real" with them as well as with himself. After a lifetime of pain and all kinds of quick-fixes, Barry was taking a new path of honesty, spirituality, wisdom, and sincerity. Barry's courage, leadership, and emerging radiance touched my heart. His story and very presence were a testament to the strength of the group's support, the fellowship of the 12-step meetings, and all the conditions that contributed—against all odds—to turning Barry's life around.

I directly experienced the light in Barry's eyes and the depth of joy in his heart. The opportunity to share in his journey was a blessing or spiritual experience for both of us, and I refer to his manifestation of the divine or *spirit* as *inspiring*.

Many times inspiration comes in more subtle packages than dramatic personal transformations or group advancement ceremonies. Some of our clients are walking miracles just for surviving. One individual, Alice, was one such miracle. Her attempts at living with what life handed her amounted to attending 12-step meetings, engaging in challenging relationships, getting therapy, taking medications, and pursuing spirituality. As we looked into each other's eyes, my heart reached out to her as I sensed how much she had persevered even to the extent that she could face me and ask for help. I reflected on Alice's presence and her story after the session and thought of how this woman was similar to a home in a Third-World shantytown. Alice had managed to keep herself together with baling wire, discarded metal and cardboard, chunks of debris, and pieces of wood. Some people may not have thought the home was beautiful, and the home may have difficulties withstanding severe weather; however, I was inspired. This home was built on very little foundation, and in the spirit of survival and in the midst of sometimes hostile elements, she constructed a life with whatever was immediately available. That it lasted this well and for this long was a testament to Alice's resourcefulness, continued perseverance, and courage.

Under similar circumstances, I may have folded and not had the wherewithal to persevere. Alice's story teaches me about keeping the small things in perspective and about the possibilities of resilience. Her continued quest for happiness, her ability to connect with others, and her soft, sweet smile attest to a force of creativity and love that is present in the universe.

Many clients have had difficulties and barriers more severe than Alice, yet we see our clients embody a sense of humor or a love for people or for life.

Sometimes their smile lightens our heart or we notice how they persevere even 5% of the time. They may be so hurt that they cannot trust us, yet they may become vulnerable to the tiniest degree with us in the hope that doing so will help them taste happiness. They may have been so mistreated that the world feels like a prison and they may have reinforced the prison walls with self-imposed shame, self-sabotaging behavior, or negative thoughts; yet they may possess the slightest bit of courage that allows them to begin to face these truths.

Some clients will argue with us and resist us, yet even these folks inspire us. We let ourselves be touched with the fight and energy that remains inside and we tune into how genuinely human it is to struggle against the prospect of change and to let go. In the spirit of radical acceptance, we understand that each client will interact with us in a different manner and we lovingly embrace this reality. While the person who has just beaten her children is willing to make eye contact, we are inspired by the part of her—however small—that is willing to face the reality of what has occurred.

In the midst of our inspiration, clients experience that practitioners do not loathe them in the way that they perhaps loathe themselves or in the way that others have shamed them. We marvel at their strengths, and we give clients a sense that their journeys—embedded with courage and resolve—are uplifting for us. Clients, then, begin to internalize a mirrored image that includes sacredness and love. This image slowly replaces ever-so-common client stories that are clouded with self-loathing. That is the healing power that our inspiration has.

Inspiration is important food that enables us as practitioners to carry out our strong back, soft front work. We return to our clients with a smile on our face and energy to engage because each time we see movement we are nurtured. Our heart opens wide and we are better able to hold the client's and the world's pain during difficult times.

This chapter focuses on how we engage in skillful caring. We discussed the importance of curiosity, presence, compassion, and cultural awareness as well as the importance of developing willingness and competence regarding taking responsive action—for example, cleaning our bowl. When we allow our clients' lives to touch our hearts and inspire us, we mutually establish a healing environment beneficial to ourselves as practitioners and to our clients.

# Chapter Six

# BEARING WITNESS TO TRAUMA AND PAIN

*Beyond Clinical Distance*

*And what does it mean to be a murdered young girl, her mother, her killer, the killer's mother, a policeman? It means that at that moment there is not separation between that person and me. In Zen practice, . . . our minds become more . . . spacious, with less attachment to any ideas and preconceptions about who we are.*

—Bernie Glassman

*I feel the despair . . . (and) . . . I always resist. I guess that's why it's called despair. If you went willingly, it would be called something helpful, like purification or renewal. Its staring defeat and annihilation in the face that's so terrifying. . . . But I've come to trust it deeply. It's enriched my life and taught me not to fear the dark.*

—Darlene Cohen

Years ago, I was in El Salvador in the aftermath of the Truth Commission. People throughout the country were beginning to tell their stories of the tragic, traumatic, and gruesome things that had happened directly to them, or that they had witnessed and somehow lived to tell about. Some of the in-print narratives painted images so disturbing that the memories are with me today, some 20 years later. Additionally, I heard first-person accounts from El Salvadorans of torture and brutal acts of rape and violence both in El Salvador and in Chicago, where many El Salvadorans had settled.

97

I knew very little then about what to do when I was in the presence of a person telling me what had happened to them. I sensed that I could not erase what had happened to them nor could I explain away the dramatic events that would forever change their lives. I attempted to offer my presence and to listen with all my heart. In some way, I would feel the pain along with those suffering, and I would express, in one form or another, the grief that they themselves were either feeling or were too numb to feel. I probably offered "smart" advice too often and was somewhat disconnected from the reality of these traumatized individuals.

In recent times, I sit with clients and with the world's pain in a manner that is referred to as *bearing witness*. Bearing witness epitomizes strong back, soft front work in that it demands solidity and stillness of mind as well as a heart that may be broken while in the presence of suffering. I enter situations with clients or communities and open to the reality that the unfolding experience is unpredictable and the outcome is out of my control. The elements that act as a container for the client and me are: (a) the honest self-acknowledgment that I do not know — which creates space and nonreactivity; (b) the intention to listen deeply and be touched and to participate in the sacred shared experience of storytelling or the unfolding of events; (c) the disposition to not place myself above anyone.

Before I see a client for the first time, I may have some background information on the client either from an intake form or from a file. As I look through the material and familiarize myself with who this person may be, I begin to construct a tentative story — or to sound more scientific — a tentative hypothesis about key dynamics in this person's life. Perhaps I need to find out more about this. Maybe intervention X or Y will be helpful. We are mindful of not falling in love with our speculations, hypotheses, or projections; however, as mentioned in Chapter 5's sections regarding diverse populations, such thinking can prime the pump to allow us to move out of our familiar deluded state where our narrow thinking and ignorance colors the information we receive.

We read the intake from a client, John, who reveals some of the most horrific abuse one could imagine, and we assume that his brokenheartedness and early-age drug addiction were most deeply rooted in these experiences. We begin to think that we know the reason John initially appeared in the substance abuse agency. We later learn, however, in the course of John's treatment, that losing his first child to SIDS precipitated his heaviest and riskiest drug use, and when he read his autobiography during his treatment group, he was most emotional while reviewing his son's death rather than his own abuse history. We come to understand that we did not truly know this client at all when we started working with him and we did not precisely know what events meant to him. We think we know him a little better now; however, we may ask ourselves whether he feels safer to grieve over the loss of his child than over humiliating abuse suffered at the hands of his female caretaker. We wonder if this is the reason that he will allow himself to address his son's SIDS death rather than the abusive events that we assume led to his PTSD. Does it even matter whether expressing grief over losing his child is safer or more important? To what degree will processing grief in either realm contribute to or compromise recovery *for this individual?*

I entered a relationship with this client in a space of not knowing with an accompanying realization that certainty was unachievable. Even as we begin to know a client a little bit better, we still do not know. As we bear witness, we embrace not knowing. Our intention is to do the best that we can. We rely on a recipe with the following ingredients: being grounded in the moment and guided by the moment (letting the moment speak to us in the same manner Martin Luther King let God speak to him), utilizing knowledge that we have accumulated and, most of all, hearing and incorporating words of wisdom from the client about what is effective. The proportions in this recipe change from client to client; thus the precise recipe for engagement and intervention is also unknown. Ultimately, bearing witness as it pertains to helping practitioners means we come face to face with the reality that we carry out our work in the midst of what First Nation's People refer to as the "Great Mystery," and we do not grasp for so-called knowledge or formulas in order to shrink from or compensate for working in the unknown.

This manner of entering and working in the unknown is rooted in the physical/mindful process of tuning into the breath. As Darlene Cohen (2000) discusses, there is a significant difference between "breath-based" or "label-based" practitioners. While doing breath-based work, we solidly take our seat in a climate of compassion with no particular agenda or outcome in mind. We keep ourselves grounded and calm and notice as our judgments arise and pass through. Bearing witness is more aligned with "breath-based" work.

While engaged in label-based helping, we generate stories and entertain all kinds of concepts that attempt to explain the individual in the room with us. We become averse to not-knowing and strive to conceptualize and categorize. At times, this categorization can have some utility, but engaging in this manner often has the deleterious effects of reducing our intimacy with the client — because we see the individual through a stereotyping lens — and devaluing, or as Patrick Corrigan (2007) discussed, stigmatizing the individual.

The second principle relates to the importance of listening deeply and being touched while sharing the experience with the client. The notion of "sharing the experience" from a Zen perspective is different than that which is discussed within a traditional helping profession paradigm. According to Joan Halifax, when we bear witness, we allow ourselves to experience the *boundlessness* of the story: the suffering, the despair, and the threads of joy and the humor. The sun is our beating heart, and the story and the suffering, the emotion and the trauma are ours—client and practitioner. As Bernie Glassman (1998) wrote:

> [W]hen we listen, when we really pay attention to the sound of joy and suffering in the universe, then we are not separate from them, we become them. Because in reality we are not separate from those who suffer. We are them; they are us. (p. 78)

The spirit of this boundless nature of existence relates to the third principle of bearing witness—that the practitioner is not above the client. Although I may have a diploma on my wall, although I may have an agency badge, although I may have more formal education and more social status, I am not any better than my clients. This statement may sound ludicrous in its simplicity, but let us be brutally honest: What kinds of jokes do some of us make about clients? Who sits in the comfortable office chair and who sits in the cheaper office furniture? Who is slapped with labels and characterizations that none of us would tolerate for even a moment? Whose life is characterized and labeled through the misdeeds and failures that brought them into the service environments and who is the professional, paid helper? When we bear witness, we see them as us and us as them. There is no superior-inferior and we witness our judgments as passing waves of thought and not as reality.

## BEARING WITNESS TO OUR LIVES

A current example illustrates what it means to bear witness. I briefly checked the Internet before writing, and today found there was the usual sensational story highlighted in an opening screen of one of the Internet service providers. A man had mugged a 101-year-old woman and there was video footage available for the curious. I nearly always decide to bypass this kind of toxic sensationalism that I believe has the effect of demoralizing people while offering little benefit. This time I decided to watch the video because this video would depict a sad but real event in a world that I am not separate from and, as a person writing about bearing witness, it would be incongruent for me to shy away from watching.

I indicated with a click of the mouse that I wished to watch the video and could feel my heart beat a bit faster in anticipation. Predictably, a commercial appeared; footage of this woman's beating was going to be used to make money for the ISP and to increase patronage of a video/DVD distributor. Finally, the footage appeared and actually served as backdrop for a reporter's expressed outrage and her brief interview with an expert on "matters like this." The video showed a man approaching an older woman, hitting her twice in the face, taking her purse, and pushing her to the ground before leaving on his bicycle. The video was shown five or six times while the "reporter" expressed disgust and wonderment at how this could happen. The expert countered that the perpetrator probably lived nearby and had sociopathic tendencies. His analysis lasted for 10 seconds or so. The reporter summarized her frustration with the hope that when the perpetrator finally gets locked up, his fellow prisoners will teach him about hurting an old lady. The expert smiled and the video report ended.

Bearing witness to this video report meant that I became connected to the woman who was victimized. I have been victimized; I have had tragic things come into my life that I have not asked for; I have felt powerless. I have felt the pain of others who have suffered. I do not know what pain from this event is like for her; but I live in the river of pain with her. I am sorry that the world's violence has taken her as a victim; and because she was a victim and people around the world are victims, we are all victims. Bearing witness for this still-nameless human being means that I experience whatever arises. I let myself be moved, and being moved means that my heart moves and eventually my body moves. I may respond by taking a deep breath, writing a letter to the woman, or participating in a peace march.

Bearing witness to the event meant bearing witness to the attacker and his actions. I allowed myself to feel sadness about him, and I contemplated on how, with his one precious life, he has somehow found himself hitting an elderly woman and pushing her to the ground. Is his life so bad that he thinks these acts will make him happy? If he is sociopathic, as the expert suggests, what kinds of abuse and humiliation has he endured to get to the point where his alienation from the world is so complete? I know people who have suffered such indignities, humiliation, and daily violence that this kind of behavior is understandable. How damaged can his moral compass be that he is so lost in this world? I have some sense of having a faulty moral compass. Although there is major tragedy going on all over the world, getting this book published preoccupies me more than nearly anything else happening in the world. I routinely eat out at nice restaurants and spend enough on a meal to feed 20 people for a day. I bemoan the cowardice and opportunism of our politicians, yet I have written few letters to Congress. No, I have not punched and pushed a 101-year-old woman, but maybe I would if I had lived this man's life. What about soldiers who shoot civilians under the massive stress of combat? How would I act if I were one of the soldiers? What about single mothers who beat their seemingly impossible-to-control children? Bearing witness is about sitting in the middle of it all with the intention not to judge. Judgments, however, will arise and then our intention is to be honest with what is arising and not get sucked into our concepts about who people are, and how worthy or unworthy they are.

What about the news reporter, her dramatic reporting and her wish that the perpetrator get a good lesson in prison? Is she truly passionate about the victimized woman? Are she, the ISP, and the advertiser just selling violence and despair? What about me for writing about all of this in this book? How am I different from the reporter or the ISP? What are my motives?

All of these questions are rhetorical. As a frequent practitioner in bearing witness, I no longer run through lists like these in order to help me connect to the universal nature of actions, experiences, and traumas. Before watching this video, I breathed deeply and prepared to enter the territory of the unknown. I allowed myself to experience connectedness with the entire land-scape: the woman, the mugger, the reporter, the expert, the people working for the ISP, and the people involved with the advertising company. We all suffer from delusion, opportunism, small-mindedness, and violence. Eventually, intimacy with this reality—as well as the reality involving universal joy and love—becomes the ground of our work while we are bearing witness.

## BEARING WITNESS WITH CLIENTS

When we are intimate with our clients, we do not get lost in our thoughts and do not seek to entertain ourselves by wishing that things were other than they are. We hold our seat and do not engage the mind with frenetic energy related to making sure this separate being—"practitioner"—formulates the right words in order to help the other being—"client." In the midst of this kind of energy, we may run through our conceptualizations of who the client is, how we may or may not help, whether we are good enough or appear competent. This diarrhea of words and concepts separates us from the painting that we and the client are developing while we sit together.

Bearing witness is about letting go of notions regarding clinical processes. Psychiatrist Richard Mollica (2006) found that when he collected oral histories from traumatized Cambodian women, the stories that emerged were rich, freely given, and healing—more so than when he engaged in traditional clinical relationships with them. Narratives had a consistent structure that involved the reporting of facts—often in meticulous detail—and grappling with the social context and personal meaning of the traumatic experiences.

Recently, a woman who was diagnosed with PTSD told me of the enormous healing power involved in reading her trauma-laced autobiography to a treatment group. She reported that while the client group and practitioners were doing nothing but bearing witness to her and her story, she, for the first time in her life, was not experiencing shame regarding the many horrific events that she had lived through. Holding the space in silence—with no clever commentary, analysis, or ideas about what to do next—created a container of sacredness, acceptance, and personal well-being that would not have necessarily occurred had there been interpretations, suggestions, and significant mental activity of other participants in the room. During the reading, the words were "taken out of" the people in the room, allowing the storyteller to paint, with relative freedom, the canvas with her life narrative.

A similar dynamic exists inside the halls of 12-step meetings. Professionals are suspicious, and perhaps insecure, regarding the manner by which healing occurs because the meetings' process does not involve any words or special knowledge of professionals or designated experts. In a space of nonjudgment, people share their stories and listen with their hearts. They attain wisdom, become honest and self-aware, and develop self-acceptance in an environment where they do not get verbal feedback. More precise insight or understanding is reserved for times when the sponsor provides direct verbal feedback. The manner in which a sponsor's interventions complement the 12-step meetings themselves is parallel to the way in which the practitioner's bearing witness is eventually supplemented by other kinds of interventions. We discuss how bearing witness *incorporates practitioner action*; thus, it involves more than passive observation suggested by the term *witness*.

## CONTEMPLATION EXERCISE

Think of a client who inspires you or is memorable. Slightly close your eyes and begin to breathe slowly and deliberately. Bring your attention to your abdomen as it rises and falls/expands and contracts. Bring an image of your client into your heart and start listening to his or her story. Notice that as the story progresses, your attention may wander and, with your breath, bring your concentration back to the client. Watch as any theorizing or categorizing occurs and let these thoughts go, returning to the

*(Continued)*

essence of your client, his or her described life, and your open heart. *Let yourself be touched by your client and his or her story.* Appreciate the universal nature of the story and the ways in which we are all sharing the story's events and consequences. Stay in this space for a while, letting the sense of what to do (how to intervene) come to you. Do not seek answers regarding what to do or what the outcome is supposed to look like.

## DEVELOPING A SPACIOUS HEART TO HOLD PAIN

When I can be the witness,
all manner of miracles occur—
old wounds heal, the past
reveals itself to be released,
present dramas play themselves
out without sinking emotional
talons into my soft skin. The
witness welcomes truth and
dares to meet reality on its
own terms. It is the ground
in which the seeds of
transformation take root
and finally flower. When
the witness is awake, the
lake of mind is still, and
in that mirrored surface,
I see my own true face as
Spirit smiling back at me.
—**Danna Faulds**

How do we hold the pain of our loved ones, our clients, or our students without becoming, debilitated, chronically depressed, alienated, or angry? These feelings at times seem to solidify as either compassion fatigue or vicarious traumatization. Practitioners need to develop commitment to monitor our level of mental health and to send ourselves compassion in the midst of distress. Practitioners may respond that this kind of admonition is oppressive. "Not only am I failing with my clients, but I am also failing by not doing things like going to the gym or going for walks in nature!" It is easy to develop the mentality that taking care of yourself is frivolous or a bourgeois add-on for people who are self-absorbed and perhaps less dedicated to helping others.

Effective helping, however, demands self-care from the outset. Many professional books and texts discuss things like burnout prevention with a list of possible ways of ameliorating stress and gaining satisfaction in a manner that reinforces the notion that self-care is an endeavor pursued in the hours after the job. This kind of discussion proceeds from the dualistic foundation that practitioners are engaged with taking care of others at the job and are taking care of themselves at home. With that logic, there would appear to be virtually no self-care opportunities for caregivers who are home bound with people receiving their help.

The Zen approach to bearing witness means that we move beyond the work-home duality and consistently bear witness to our own—the helper's—process. We face trauma and pain in the spirit of nondenial, and we actively create space in which we can hold it all. Creating space means that we let the pain penetrate our being and consciously let go of grasping it and ruminating over it. We see violence and victimization for what it is and we are honored that we are able to experience the richness of the client's life. We celebrate our intention to contribute through witnessing, and we realize that sitting with pain provides lessons and opportunities.

We create space through not pushing anything away and through settling into the reality that this story is surrounded by universal love or spirit. Some of us may contemplate that the universe, some higher purpose, or God transcends the particular story, and some of us may pray. We send love to our clients and people we are caring for, and we do the best we can to cultivate joy and to have our joy be a gift to all humanity.

Our clients rely on our buoyancy and sense of well-being while we are present with them. To some extent, we do "gas-up" while we are home and away from the fray of intensive caregiving, counseling, social work, or teaching. We do cultivate other parts of our lives to enhance the store of resources available when we meet our clients. However, it is important not to have the moments *with* clients turn into times when the reserves of the heart are depleted and drained dry. Being with others exercises the heart as we generously give our presence. Being present may nurture us and build on our capacities to effectively serve.

Even in the midst of paperwork or staff meetings, we find ways to take care of ourselves so we do not burn out. We light a candle as we do our paperwork, we briefly imagine the smiling face of our client, or we cheerfully and enthusiastically recite the words of John Kabat-Zinn (1990), "Time to live the whole catastrophe NOW!"

Everything discussed here still may not work. We find ourselves more and more depleted even though we have been bearing witness to ourselves as well as our clients. We generously honor ourselves and do not send blame or shame to our pain. Perhaps we need to retreat into the relative world of self and administer self-kindness and direct—away from the client—self-care. We stand back, set clear boundaries, and heal our heart and mind. At the point of vicarious traumatization, the cracks in the shells of your clients are becoming your cracks and you need time and strategies to patch them up. When you feel rejuvenated, you make a pact with yourself regarding how you maintain your open-heartedness and mental health. Then you re-enter the world of your clients.

The amount of time away may not be as important as its quality. It could be a week-long vacation, a weekend, an evening at home, or 5 quiet, meditative minutes in the car. Connecting with joy and calmness and the bigger spiritual picture is valuable medicine to maintain our spacious heart.

## TELLING ALL AND HIDING ALL

We bear witness to a contradictory dynamic expressed by Judith Herman (1997) that is often profound in the case of traumatized clients and sometimes present for other clients as well. Many people who have had major life difficulties secretly wish for the opportunity to share their stories with someone who will listen and not judge. It is healing to share one's inner life with another. People who have suffered sometimes feel as though their experience sets them apart from the living; the sufferers, thus, sense that they are otherworldly. When a witness compassionately sees the unwatchable and believes the unbelievable, the storyteller may feel that she is connected to the witness and the witness's very presence because the individual may communicate that she (the storyteller) is worthy of being heard and seen. Additionally, denial of life and what has occurred is often a coping strategy for the traumatized individual. The antidote to denial is most complete when the trauma survivor comes out of herself or himself and shares about her or his inner life and experiences. It is one thing to tell yourself about things that have happened, and sometimes this discussion exists in a context of perpetual rumination, perseveration, and self-castigation. It is still another to engage another human being in the trauma narrative.

In a similar vein, the fifth step in 12-step recovery programs involves the participant's sharing his or her "personal inventory" with another person. It is powerful to become honest with yourself and sincerely explore personal characteristics and events, which is the fourth step; however, this power is enhanced and further healing is mobilized when the fourth-step work—usually a written narrative—is shared with another. The process of sharing and actually facing our difficulties is the fifth step: *We admitted to our higher power, to ourselves, and to another human being the exact nature of our wrongs.* In this sharing, the listener holds some of the story about the person's life and shortcomings. The story becomes just that—a story—and events, mistakes, and trauma become less tightly wound around the narrator. In the course of sharing, the individual perhaps begins a process of coming to peace with and feeling less overwhelmed by life's difficult or tragic circumstances. At this point, the participant has not only sought the truth about her life, she has provided herself an antidote to denial, dissociation, or numbing through recruiting and involving witnesses to her personal story—her higher power, herself, and another individual.

## Humiliation and Vulnerability

Mollica (2006) discusses that humiliation, however, is so embedded in many traumatized individuals' psyches, that as much as the person has an instinct to share and receive the benefits of sharing, an oppositional force related to the client's deep sense of humiliation and shame forces the narrative underground. As practitioners, part of our effort relates to our bearing witness to the inherent conflict that people have regarding how much they will tell us:

> Enigmatically, the state of humiliation seems relatively easy to create despite the victim's loathing for the perpetrator or rejection of the perpetrator's goals and values. Why human beings are easily susceptible to humiliation is unclear, but whatever the reasons, this inherent tendency toward fragility and emotional vulnerability makes the job of the perpetrator much easier. (p. 74)

Ultimately, Mollica continues, humiliation and shame go underground because many traumatized people have a deep fear of being rejected for who they are and what they have experienced. It is thus relatively easy for us as practitioners to be feared as potentially rejecting and to be experienced as contributing to the client's heightened sense of vulnerability and shame.

A recent group example illustrates the vulnerability to being exposed that some clients experience. One woman, Juanita, was checking in about how her week had been going. She mentioned various struggles related to her housing situation, visitation with her children who had been placed in foster care, and the instability of her relationship with her boyfriend. I listened patiently and calmly, and I felt moved hearing Juanita's story, though she herself displayed little emotion. As we will see next, part of bearing witness also involves taking action; thus, I mentioned to her that she seemed like she was "barely hanging on," and I wondered aloud how life could be any better for her—a solution-focused question. Immediately, from across the room another woman confronted me for not just leaving Juanita alone and for playing mind games with her. She argued that it should be enough for a person so vulnerable to tell the group about her difficulties and not have to hear me reflect on how she is "hanging on" nor have to answer questions about how things could get better. Another person nodded her agreement, while a male group member joined the chorus critiquing my involvement and claimed that I sometimes pressed too hard to get people to talk about things they did not want to talk about.

Juanita expressed that she felt cared for when I reflected on my sense of her struggle and explored ways that life could become better. I calmly told the group that my intention was never to play mind games with people and that there was often ambivalence regarding talking: an urge to be open about what was going on and a simultaneous tug to hold back. It made sense to me that people would get uneasy and even angry when it looked like I was being invasive and insensitive. In the spirit of bearing witness, I discussed all this without malice or any sense of trying to defend myself or prove others wrong. The pain of vulnerability and powerlessness was in the room and it was my pain, too. I appreciated what it meant to feel vulnerable and joined with the group members.

I was passionate, however, about communicating to the group members that my intentions never involve trying to hurt people. I believe group members sensed my love for them as I spoke. Soon one group member after another discussed how they often had held back, whether in individual counseling or in the group, and how the experience of being pushed had yielded some great results. The male client who had agreed previously that my "head games" sometimes went too far then talked about how his relationship with his wife had improved greatly after another group leader and I pushed him to address his struggles in this arena.

The issue of being violated by overly invasive social workers, counselors, psychologists, nurses, and doctors exists for all individuals. People who have already suffered violations may be especially vigilant and feel quite threatened in the face of practitioner inquiries. Such responses speak even further to the value of bearing witness to people's pain and vulnerabilities. At times, it is fruitful to risk reaching out and exploring difficult subjects; then the task becomes bearing witness to the reactions and responses that arise from these kinds of interventions. As well, we may bear witness to the no-win choice that we seem to be left with at times: between effectively keeping the peace and colluding with the clients to not raise *anything* threatening, taboo, or vulnerable. We similarly bear witness to our own reluctance to step into the unknown where people may feel hurt or frightened but where important growth awaits.

We are respectful and committed to maximizing safety and not doing harm; however, we do not assume that clients with extremely difficult pasts will all respond the same way in our presence. We must be prepared for the possibility that our casual reliance on standard interventions may not suit our clients well and that bearing witness to fear, vulnerability, mistrust, and eventually client narratives may be necessary to work effectively.

## BEARING WITNESS AND RESPONSE-ABILITY

Engaging with Juanita over her personal struggles and engaging with the group over their sense of Juanita's being invaded were part of the bearing witness process. This process involves deep listening and observing, as well as a willingness to enter uncertainty and face and become intimate with what is truly there. Bearing witness also entails a nonreactive response. Sometimes the response involves using a pillow to gently prop up the head of a bedridden person in a hospice setting, sometimes it involves advocating on behalf of a client, sometimes it involves a counseling intervention, and sometimes it involves staying quiet.

We come to an awareness that we need to have the ability to respond, which is also to say we have responsibility. From a Zen perspective, responsibility derives from the inherent connection we all have to one another and our essential nonseparateness that we discussed in earlier chapters. We are "response-able" for the world in the spirit of the famous 1985 song entitled "We Are the World." This song called for the world "to come together as one" and make the choice to give on behalf of people in Africa suffering from starvation. The subtle difference from the Zen perspective is that the world is *already* together as one, but often we are not awake to this reality. Regardless of orientation, the call to respond as one—and recognize that we are response-able—is what is important. Implicit in this call is the sense that one individual and the whole are not separate: "It's true we make a better day just you and me." (See USA for Africa, 1985.)

Thus, we act with a degree of conviction and sense of buoyancy because our actions are being supported by the rest of the universe. We are acting with the intention to make the world better, whether we are changing a diaper, smiling to someone, donating money, providing service, or seeking social change. Our responsibility, however, does not equate with blameworthiness for what does not go well. Therefore, we do not need to feel the compulsion to say, "I am not responsible for that."

This kind of orientation regarding universal responsibility to others is sometimes alien to us. Additionally, it seems that we would be overwhelmed and rendered useless if we truly lived this way. We can imagine our boundaries under assault and our sense of personal integrity in great peril should we take on the world's pain.

## BOUNDLESSNESS AND BOUNDARIES

In the past 2 days, the pain of a particular client as well as my own daughter has been overwhelming. Personally following the idealistic advice of bearing witness and joining the boundless world of each one's suffering has left me in a state of despair. My client is a 20-year-old woman trying to maintain custody of her high-need, colicky child while living with an unsupportive mother who used to take my client to drug houses with her throughout her childhood. Additionally, my client confesses that she is having strong cravings to use, feels that her life is going nowhere, has already lost one child to Child Protective Services, has trouble sleeping, has no money, and constantly deals with traumatic events and relationships that haunt her. Meanwhile, my daughter has been battling hallucinations that have been more acute over the past few days. I daily experience the wounds of her schizophrenia, which was diagnosed 1.5 years ago. She tells me how she is acutely aware of her declining memory and impaired functioning, and her startling and horrific nightmares have kept us both up over the past couple of nights.

In this case, I bear witness to my own despair. At first, as Darlene Cohen's (2000) opening quote suggests, I resist. I do not want to go to this dark place but part of its call suggests that there are no options here. I could choose to escape or engage in denial; however, I have come to trust that I must face the darkness. As I stop to feel what is happening, I realize that I need to embrace the relative world in the process of bearing witness as well. Yes, my daughter's pain and my client's pain are my pain, as Bernie Glassman (1998) suggested earlier; however, I also need to maintain boundaries and commit myself to personal health and happiness.

As we discuss more thoroughly in the next chapter, I embrace the Middle Way between the apparent dualities of boundaries and boundlessness. Ultimately, from the view of absolute reality, the client, my daughter, and I all share the universe's pain—it belongs to no one being or nobody. When I live here, I allow my client's and my daughter's suffering to touch my soft front and open heart. In a sense, it is our suffering—the suffering of the universe. An example from clinical supervision brings home the importance of this absolute or big picture view. One clinical trainee has increasingly revealed various difficulties and traumas that he has endured throughout his life. As he has told particular stories, he came to realize how hard he has worked to avoid experiencing humiliation and how this avoidance has led him to be a taskmaster with his clients to the degree that he has become unempathic at times. His rigid, strong back has served him in his climb to move forward in spite of severe barriers, and his strong back currently enables him to get things done and be a model for his clients. Unfortunately, because he had been closed off to his own pain, he was less able to access and open to the pain of others. Until this time, he has not so much lived in the boundlessness of the feelings and stories and lives of his clients.

I, on the other hand, lean more in the direction of boundlessness regarding clients or family members. One apparent example is the manner in which this book is written. My family's struggles enter the book and I enter the book—failures and all. You as the reader see me and you experience the struggles and pain that I have. I do not own this pain as my own and invite you to identify with me and share my hurts.

Though I am adept at bearing witness and holding the struggles of others, I am less skillful at setting limits and working with the boundaries of "I and thou" found in the relative world. A sense of these boundaries allows us to be skillful and balanced about what we take on and, as helpers, we are better able to demonstrate trust in "the other" to find her way and become empowered. Clients feel safe with solid practitioner-client boundaries because they sense that they do not have to deal with the practitioner's problems, that the helping environment is predictable and not emotionally abusive, and that they can focus on their own betterment without the contamination of the helper's personal agenda or baggage. Helper boundaries also create a clear field for practitioner health and life apart from the world of the client or struggling family member.

Residing in a world of boundaries allows me to honor my commitment to be personally joyful. Although joy is a boundless state, when I embody joy, I am prepared to give gifts to my clients, my daughter, and the universe. Embodying joy and internal peace allows me to be an instrument of help in a world of so much suffering, anxiety, and discord.

While embracing personal boundaries, I reflect on my personal life and permit myself to feel compassion for my struggles. I hold my dilemmas with patience and an open heart, and I begin to cultivate a sense of appreciation for elements not related to my pain and eventually for the pain itself. I come to realize that I do not have control over the experiences or the suffering of others, and in doing so, I release attachments to imagined outcomes. Although I am able to respond to the universe, I develop clarity between response-ability and control. I become keenly aware of how the ground of my interactions with others is about entering the unknown, being a nonreactive witness to what is, calming my judgments, and responding without attachments to imagined outcomes. I simultaneously hold the soft front disposition regarding the interconnectedness of everyone's pain and joy as well as the strong back posture of clear boundaries.

How do boundaries and boundlessness play out in the way I relate to my young, drug-addicted client as well as with my own daughter? In each case, I experience their pain and their sense of the world as closing in on them. Although their situations sometimes make their respective tunnels particularly dark, they are mere poster children for universal difficulties related to biological, psychological, and social causes and conditions. As I mentioned earlier, my daughter's and my client's pain became my pain, which became the world's pain and I found myself in despair. Developing the stance of *witness*, however, began the process of not so much identifying with pain, and the pain became less solid and all-encompassing. There was an "I" in witness that allowed me to shake free and develop a perspective related to boundaries as well as one related to boundlessness.

## OH CRAP, NOW WHAT?

My son's early childhood behavior and developmental issues led to frustration and hundreds of incidents of *oh crap, now what?* When he yelled in the car because he missed seeing the dinosaur statue on the side of Route 80 between Sacramento and San Francisco, the destruction of our fragile familial equilibrium seemed complete. His distress took over his entire body and sense of well-being. His sister lovingly attempted to soothe him, the volume inside the car soared, and my wife and I tried to remain calm and sane and keep the car on the road. My wife and I developed abilities over time to bear witness to it all. In the midst of frequent tantrums or distress, we would witness that moment of *oh crap, now what*, and how it was a jolt to our reality. A tightening of the stomach, a sense of disease in the chest, and overall disorientation would strike. These moments offered rich tastes of despair and inclinations of curling up into a ball and giving up, fleeing the scene immediately, or gravitating toward rage fueled by utter helplessness.

The main thread of *oh crap, now what* has always been a deep sense of uncertainty. The first part of the uncertainty relates to confusion about what actually is taking place. *Now what* in this case means—what is hitting me now or just what is it that I am facing? Witnessing child or adolescent anger or rage, hearing a *DSM* diagnosis for a child, being in the middle of struggles related to school or peers were all times when I felt that sense of being knocked across the head. There was a moment of disorientation and, again, that sense of *what just hit me?* The same kind of feeling occurs when we are with clients. A new crisis arises (I thought we just worked through this issue), the depth of someone's trauma is meaningfully revealed for the first time, deep dissatisfaction is revealed about the helping process, or a group becomes totally disruptive. Imagine yourself identifying with the following while you are breathing slowly and calmly:

> I am in the middle of a confusing swirl of emotions, stories, and behaviors, and the outcome is completely uncertain. My calm breathing becomes the ground in the midst of the tumultuous moment. I begin to *see clearly* which addresses the first riddle embedded in *now what*. What I see is that I have no immediate answers, that the chaos and pain is okay as chaos and pain, that I am compassionate toward all parties involved including myself, and, if I stay grounded in the moment, I will be response-able and engage in an action or series of actions that will represent my best efforts (and perhaps these efforts will fail).

The second twist of *now what* involves the question, "What do I/we *do* now?" Most of the doing relates to applying the brakes to reactive, quick-fix responses that often come more from the helper's desire to halt the troublesome behaviors, attitudes, or emotions or from the helper's need for ego gratification than from the commitment to a process that connects to meaningful and satisfying action. Strikingly, even in the midst of crisis, *now what* takes us into the doing realm of maintaining our collaborative relationship and respect for the other. The medium of this work, as Harlene Anderson (1997) advocates, is dialog that provides the ground of liberation from "the authoritarian claims of those-who-are-in-the-know" (p. 108). In other words, what we *do* is honest, authentic, nonauthoritarian engagement. What we do is enter into the fray with a willingness to be vulnerable along with our client, student, or family member, and to the greatest extent possible, mutually discover the right steps to take. As we are involved in the doing part of *now what*, we are aware of how we may be criticized for our inadequate participation or the degree to which we have not been helpful. We embrace that possibility and welcome that sentiment if it should arise. Our only decision at this point involves whether to invite the question of the client's responsibility when an outcome is experienced as unsatisfactory.

In Zen, we embrace the *now what* moments as they arise. Reb Anderson suggests saying "thank you" to whatever comes up with the understanding that infinite causes and conditions created it, and that there was "no alternative" to how that moment unfolded. Joan Halifax describes how she embraces being in the wilderness (Halifax, 1993), literally and figuratively—in other words, to be "bewildered" is an opportunity for growth and awakening. But before we become too enamored with hanging out in a state of bewilderment, we must realize that clients, students, and others whom we are helping are counting on our presence, clarity, and, at times, concrete directed efforts. Therefore, we spend enough time in the wilderness (bewildered) only to be aware, that to some extent, we are there. We do not have the perfect answers for those whom we serve; their pain and our own pain disturb us and throw us off balance; resource deficiencies and personal and societal barriers seem insurmountable; we are not sure how much to do for others, how much to do with others, or how much not to do; people's anger and despair frighten us or temporarily paralyze us.

We must not react to our bewilderment with action undertaken merely to act. When we act with this kind of reactivity, we do so because we are scared of the wild and scared to let others see how scared we are. Instead of reactive action, we return to our authentic selves and let ourselves be fearful of the wilderness. Though we are fearful, we are committed to staying grounded in our breath and to deliberately moving forward one step at a time. We are not necessarily sure what direction we are moving in; however, we know that our intentions are to be as helpful as possible. Helpfulness derives from our being present for the client, hearing the client's wishes, relying on knowledge about the person's situation, and being true to the structure of the helping encounter. We walk one step at a time through the forest with a compass that has some degree of utility. Because we walk *with* our helpee, we gain in the conviction that our journey will bear fruit. Eventually, fear is replaced with a quiet strength that permeates the helper's being in the form of total acceptance for walking in the wilderness of uncertainty.

One clinical supervisee, Mary, who worked at a foster family agency, discussed a case in which her bearing witness did not lead to skillful responseability. A well-respected foster father asked Mary to be present at a meeting that became emotionally charged. The foster father envisioned that during this meeting he would reveal to his 15-year-old foster child Danny that he would no longer be able to care for him. In addition to the foster family agency caseworker (Mary), the foster child's therapist was present. Because the boy had such an extensive history of acting-out and instability, the foster father had assumed that Danny would have a nonchalant or, at least, not particularly intense response to the news that he had to leave the home. Instead Danny responded with disbelief, desperation, and a broken heart. "I thought I was getting better," he said. He had some connection with his foster care siblings as well as the foster father's biological child, and Danny had adjusted to the neighborhood school. The foster father was not going to budge in his decision. He had rehearsed for this meeting for weeks.

While Danny sank into despair and withdrew from the adults around him, Danny's foster father mentioned that he had to leave the meeting in order to pick up one of the children. The two professionals were left to awkwardly deal with Danny's enormous pain. The foster family agency worker, Mary, looked at Danny's therapist for clues about what to do or what to say, but the therapist appeared to be lost. Mary did not want to step on the toes of the therapist but wanted to reach out to Danny. She asked him a couple of routine questions but soon realized that her efforts were inadequate.

Mary stated to me that at first she found herself tongue-tied and noticed how much she experienced Danny's devastation at the meeting. She also conveyed the nature of his broken heart and how the depth of his response caught everyone, including herself, off guard. She noted how awkward it was to be with Danny's therapist who seemed overwhelmed. Overall, Mary has outstanding ability when it comes to observing her own process. She was adept at bearing witness to the events and process of all that had happened; however, effective responses were not readily available to her.

Both practitioners froze in the face of the unknown. Had either one embraced her bewilderment, skillful words may have emerged. Mary may have discussed with Danny her sincere sense of not knowing what to say. This kind of remark would not involve the practitioner's motives for personal help but punctuate the truth of the pure devastation of the moment. Then the social worker or therapist could provide a container for Danny where he would not even have to talk. Danny's presence for the social worker's narrative of the events would be adequate:

> Danny, you are a wonderful person, and I am so sorry that this has happened. One of the beautiful things about you is that your heart is open, and you might think what's the point because once again you have been hurt. But this beautiful heart of yours is the reason that

people want to be with you and the reason that you do have a girl-friend who cares about you. I know that this hurts and I also know that you will pick yourself up and keep caring. I want the very best for you.

Although Danny may not have responded directly to the practitioner, he would have sensed on some level that the social worker was with him. Because of both workers' fear or unskillfulness in negotiating uncertainty, Danny, instead, experienced rejection and pain in virtual isolation.

## RIGHT SPEECH

Ultimately we walk in the wilderness with our clients; however, our accept-ance of the helping environment's wild and unpredictable nature allows us to project that we, as practitioners, have an idea about what we are doing. Our profound intention to help involves the processes of deep listening, respect, compassion for ourselves and others, and personal authenticity. We commit ourselves to right speech, one of the five precepts of Buddhism. There are useful questions to ask ourselves when seeking to determine the skillfulness of our speech with clients, students, or those receiving our help:

- Are my words truthful?
- Are my words hurtful?
- Are my words beneficial?

Sometimes our communications with people will be truthful and beneficial; however, they may hurt feelings. Sometimes we are not as sure as we initially thought regarding "the truth." Is this about truth or about my assumptions or projections. Perhaps it is better to own our words as our thoughts rather than "the truth."

With people who are readily devastated by words that sound like criticism, it may make sense to emphasize not hurting and not harming over "telling the truth." This is not to suggest that it would be helpful to lie; however, it suggests that we lean in the direction of soft nurturing more than harsh truth-telling that could add pain. Sometimes we are not clear about being benefi-cial with our words. Words that cut through the client's fog or denial may produce short-term pain and dis-ease, however they may lead to long-term benefit. Words that are truthful and lean more in the direction of creating comfort and short-term peace are perhaps not as hurtful and may produce short-term benefits; however, they may be part of helpee-practitioner collusion around not addressing difficult issues. Soft words may also be related to the practitioner's fear of client abandonment or anger.

The caretaker leans more toward unconditional acceptance and kind words. The agenda is more tilted toward acceptance and love than toward change. On the other hand, the helping professional to one degree or another dances between unconditional acceptance and amelioration of troublesome feelings, thoughts, or behavior. She or he dances back and forth between unconditional acceptance and change, emphasizing different elements of right speech at different times. Of course, it is optimal if our communication with others involves all three elements of right speech simultaneously. However, the vulnerability of the people whom we are helping means that we are often choosing between various right speech elements.

## BEARING WITNESS AND THE HELPING CULTURE

We bear witness to the lives of individuals who are dealing with many kinds of situations and who have varying degrees of opportunities, resources, openness, and skill sets to help them cope and move forward. Our helping context also affects the way in which we bear witness. In some settings, we are forced to see people in short intervals. We are encouraged in these instances to see as many people as possible and to be efficient. Sometimes the focus on this so-called efficiency means that we stop seeing the textured lives of our clients. We may be so focused on moving the client toward a particular outcome that who they are or what they have actually dealt with does not make a significant imprint on our psyche. The client, in these cases, may feel as if she is a profile of problems and deficiencies who needs to change. She is deprived of the practitioner who really "takes in" or bears witness to her life.

Sometimes, the culture of hurry or of outcome-driven work affects our commitment; other times the culture of the agency or school setting affects how much we can really allow our clients' lives to penetrate our own. One setting I am involved with provides 1 hour per week of supervision for its clinicians, 2 hours per week of group supervision for all direct service providers, and 2 hours per week of staffing time. In this setting, staff members experience that fellow staff and a clinical supervisor are bearing witness to their dilemmas with clients. These dilemmas often touch on the staff's own personal matters as well, including previous abuse history, substance abuse, relationship problems, feelings of inadequacy, and depression. Sometimes the nature of the discussions in the supervision groups—and particularly the check-ins themselves—revolve around the practitioners' life stories, triumphs, and struggles. Because there is a culture of support, practitioners at this agency are able to compassionately be there for clients in a way that I have not seen before. There is virtually no sarcastic joking about clients, there is virtually no mean-spiritedness, and there is a well of patience, good will, and dedicated service directed toward clients.

As practitioners enter group supervision time, there is a sense of a family sitting down to share the joys, trials, and tribulations of life and work. We bear witness to practitioners who may be struggling at home with a family member or confused about how to proceed with clients. Focusing on content and advice-giving occurs more often when discussing clients rather than personal matters; however, the common thread, regardless of what is being divulged, is that one person's pain is part of everyone's pain and that we are there for each other.

Despite portraying myself in this book as a spiritual, bearing-witness kind of guy, I was somewhat resistant to the degree of personal sharing that occurred during supervision group time. I picked up the previous clinical supervisor's cynicism about the extensive personal check-ins and concocted my own story about how the agency's staff was, perhaps, not so committed to their *professional* growth. Without offering reasons for my skepticism, I mentioned to the staff that I was seeking to reduce the personal check-in time. The staff held firm regarding the value of sharing their personal lives with the other staff serving as witnesses. A number of the staff were in recovery, and they argued that this kind of open-hearted, honest, and visible presentation of themselves was important for their continued sanity. They were vulnerable, they said, to relapsing. It had happened before in agency settings employing recovering addicts; this kind of sharing contributed to cultivating the rich soil that would support the staff to grow and thrive.

In fact, all people, addicts or not, are vulnerable to the challenges and stresses of life. Additionally, community building occurs when people are present not only to hear and process particular difficulties but also to celebrate triumphs and positive occurrences. In this setting, it has been a spiritual gift for the staff to come to group and rely on each other to collectively bear witness to one another's life.

In family settings or intimate home-care situations, bearing witness involves other complicated elements. It is difficult to sense boundaries when we are bearing witness to the struggles or suffering of someone in our family or someone who shares space with us. While bearing witness to the pain, uncertainty, and loss related to my daughter's schizophrenia, I bear witness to my own and my daughter's suffering. How do I help, and is my intention to "help" part of my desire to make my own life better? How do I bear witness and then go off and try to lead an out-of-family life where there is some separation from my daughter's struggles? How much do I need an objective self in order to bear witness, or is it about, as Glassman (1998) suggests, merging with the other? How do I bear witness without carrying guilt for not suffering the same maladies as my child, and how do I bear witness without being jealous or resentful of families who do not understand and/or who seem to have escaped this kind of pain? The bearing-witness dance is forever present in this kind of home situation. The reality of what Pema Chodron (1991) has coined "the wisdom of no escape" is the pervasive dynamic when living or sharing space with an individual who is suffering. As a result, we all suffer to some degree, and we learn how to embrace this reality. We see that each day is a new adventure with its own story. Some days are predominantly difficult with few bright moments and others seem to be brighter.

From a Zen perspective, we learn to courageously face what is. Our open hearts allow us to sit with what is presented and to stay present. If we constantly make a count of how long things have been bad or difficult, we will suffer more. When my son had a tantrum, I was intimate with him and with that moment. I was usually successful in not ruminating about how many times I had had to deal with this kind of behavior, nor would I let myself speculate about how many more times I could tolerate the tantrums or worry about how he may grow up. Just as one returns to the breath in meditation, whenever I found myself losing contact with my son and his distress—entertaining thoughts that led to despair or worry—I would return to the present moment and stay fresh with what was unfolding before me. I would bear witness to his distress, and my thoughts and feelings would become less important. Bearing witness in these cases meant that I was not lost in my frustration-induced judgments about how silly his tantrums were; instead, I could enter the uncertainty of the moment with a clear mind and a preparedness to help. Eventually the stories and ruminating thoughts involving the pervasiveness of the incidents, the "unfairness" of it all, and future forecasts of his life are seen for what they are—*passing thoughts*—and the reality of the moment became prominent.

In this present moment, our engagement with our clients, students, or persons for whom we are caring becomes alive. Our session or encounter reflects the true expression of our client and is not so clouded with our own story lines related to self-perceived incompetence or frustration.

## BEARING WITNESS AND NONATTACHMENT TO OUTCOME

The concept of nonattachment to outcome is confusing, particularly in a culture thoroughly infused with Western-oriented values. At first glance, it appears that if we cared about someone, we would care about how successful the person would be. If we cared about that person's success or failure, it would stand to reason that we would be emotionally invested in the attainment of particular outcomes and, therefore, emotionally and mentally affected by whether or not desirable outcomes were attained. In contrast to this kind of orientation, the notion of nonattachment to outcomes strikes one as practitioner aloofness or noncaring, or of not being on board with the mission and goals of the agency setting or the individual treatment plan.

In Zen, just as in 12-step traditions that happen to be Eastern-inspired, we recognize the degree to which we do not have control over events that occur in the universe, which include the behaviors of others. Liberation arises for us when we come face-to-face with the reality that we do not even know whether we will be alive tomorrow. What is so liberating about embracing a thought like that? It is liberating because the uncertain nature of our death is the absolute truth, and according to Zen, the more we try to hide from profound truths like these, the more we live in a world of denial and delusion. When we are able to embrace this kind of truth, we are able to live with—and in—the world as it is. We are generous to ourselves and to others about the dilemmas of life, and we begin to loosen our tight grip of identification with our beliefs and stories about what is right and about the way life should be.

As we come face-to-face with the uncertain nature of our death, we often experience some degree of fear or anxiety, and we tell the truth (to ourselves or to another) about our experience. As we come face-to-face with the uncertain nature of our client's life and whether we will have a positive impact, we tell the truth about how we do not like this reality and how it makes us feel small and unimportant. As we continue to tell the truth about these difficult realities, we begin to experience the sense that we can live in and embrace the world as it is. We accept our infinitesimal impact on the earth's affairs as Mother Teresa did when she declared that our actions are like a drop in the ocean—but oh how vital is that drop. She said, "It is not how much you do, but how much love you put into the doing that matters." Thus our point of focus in bearing witness is about maintaining our presence, engaging in nondenial, and bringing our compassion forward. Our intention, of course, is to help; however, we come face-to-face with the reality that we are not sure how to proceed and that fundamentally we have no control over the outcome.

The distinction between control and influence is important here. Control implies that action on our part leads to desired results or behaviors. At first glance, we may believe that we have this kind of control of our cars. We make adjustments as we drive along—turn our steering wheel, apply the brakes, and give the engine more or less gas. As predictable as our cars' response tends to be, further study reveals that our control is not absolute. What happens if our car is suddenly sideswiped, or we have a tire blow out, or hit a patch of ice? Suddenly the illusion of control develops a few cracks. We concede that we cannot control things like inclement weather or the behavior or performance of other drivers or all mechanical failure possibilities, but at least we maintain the illusion that we have control over ourselves.

## CONTEMPLATION EXERCISE

Who is this being who is controlling me? Is there a separate "I" who controls this "I"? What does control of one's self mean? What about if I am excessively tired or unfocused while I am on the road? Who is going to step up and control me? Is there an "I" who can intervene in a moment when I am temporarily confused about whether I am to step on the accelerator or the brake pedals? What about if my body is suffering a crisis like a heart attack? Is there still the same "I" who has control over the car?

Clearly, controlling people and their outcomes is far more complicated. Our intentions, skills, presence, and interventions are *influences* among numberless events and circumstances as well as an ecological web of causes and conditions that defy complete comprehension or description. Our attempt to control client outcomes is preposterous and we, as practitioners, would have to live in a world of denial in order to believe outcome control is operable.

When we are attached to outcomes, we are often so immersed in our own stories about how things should be that we are not adequately present for our clients. In a supervision group, one clinician revealed how frustrating and confusing her work was with a boy, Michael, who had an extensive history of being abused and neglected. It seemed that although Michael expressed his appreciation for the practitioner, the practitioner reported being frustrated, primarily with the youth's inconsistent stories and his resistance to explore his own traumatic past—one of the treatment plan's written outcomes. The practitioner's story about her own inadequate work and her frustration regarding the youth's confusing and conflicting accounts of events in his life left her feeling "overwhelmed and helpless." In fact, the practitioner had done beautiful work with Michael. Despite the boy's family credo about not trusting outsiders—which may have originated in their experience as Native Americans—the client and the practitioner had a solid, long-standing relationship. Michael was empathic with his peers in a treatment group despite being abused and neglected by family members who, for many years, were using drugs all around him. He was enjoying relative success in terms of staying out of trouble, and he was caring and loyal to his mother. Although this agency's (as well as many others') helping model involved finding the diamonds of past truths and traumas that crystallized the reasons for why the particular individual was leading a dysfunctional life, this kind of search with Michael always proved fruitless.

Bearing witness for Michael meant bearing witness to the present moment. In effect, Michael brought his past and his long-standing dilemmas into the session as he sat with the practitioner. With the Michaels of the world, we do not have to overtly talk about these experiences for us to witness what various experiences mean to them. As we bear witness to our clients' fear and humiliation, we realize that the path that our clients take to engage with us makes perfect sense. We do not judge this path as "inadequate"; instead, we embrace the degree to which we are not hearing the overt story. We see how the tiny sprouts of Michael's life have adapted and are reaching for the sun in all kinds of crooked configurations.

## LETTING GO OF OUTCOME AND PROCESS

Recently, some adolescents in an anger management group directly told me of their desire to not touch pain in their lives. Although there was an apparent level of mutual caring in the room, the youths seem disembodied—leaning and slouching in all directions and easily distracted, appearing almost as if they were seeking to be distracted. When I introduced a meditation bell to them, they settled and focused on the reverberations of the bell's beautiful sound. As they passed the bell around the room, and each of the seven boys had a chance to strike it, the room became progressively quieter and the attention to the sound more mindful. The boys were coming home to the present moment. I asked the boys to sit up straight in their seats and put their feet on the ground. "You deserve to take up space on this planet," I told them, "and putting your feet on the ground lets you connect with the world and give yourself the sense that you belong here." I added that sitting up straight was an opportunity to open their hearts and that there was no one in the room who would hurt them. The boys reflected on how unnatural it felt to even approximate this kind of posture; however, they experimented with it. Coming home to themselves through settling into the sound of the bell and experimenting with sitting up with their feet on the ground represented a *strong back, soft front* experience that seemed meaningful. Although my interaction with them was framed as a "guest" appearance, a couple of the boys asked me if I was going to return and some of them inquired about how they could get a bell. (They most likely would not have made these inquiries had they been in front of their peers on the street.)

Feeling that I was on a roll with them, I confidently approached a relaxation exercise with the group. For whatever reasons, the exercise broke down in the midst of contagious laughter, inattention, and noise. The group time was winding down and we had 5 minutes to wrap things up. "We really screwed that one up," one of the boys said and others agreed. They seemed ashamed of their behavior, as if the high quality of their earlier involvement had never happened. At that time, my heart was vast and appreciative, and I told them how much I appreciated all the risks they had taken and who they were. My life had been truly better for having met them. "Not everything works the way we would like it to," I said, "and, in fact, the falling apart of the relaxation exercise was an opportunity for me to model how to stay calm in the middle of things not turning out." Although I had a plan of activities for the group, my primary approach to being there was to bear witness to the group facilitators' (my supervisees) and the group's experience. My ground of engagement was *not knowing*—not knowing their reactions to me: a 49-year-old White guy in the midst of a diverse group of male adolescents flanked by the established leaders, two attractive females in their late 20s; not knowing their responses to having the bell passed from teen to teen (in fact up until the time the group actually began, I was not sure how I would proceed with the bell); not knowing how much to say or if the facilitators would be intimidated by my presence, and so on. I entered with an open heart and a commitment not to judge, but rather to learn. I was not better than anyone in the room. Additionally, I sensed that the moment would teach me about how to respond. Even if the response could be called a failure, and the relaxation exercise attempt would certainly qualify, I knew that I could bear witness to this failure and that the clients and I could hold that as well.

Finally, I was not attached to any particular outcome of the experience. In theory, my appearance at the group was designed to be beneficial to the supervisee, who requested my presence in order that I would gain additional insight into her work as a clinician. I was not attached to looking good in this supervisee's eyes, to having an experience where there would be no awkwardness between myself and the other facilitators, to modeling a special intervention, or to having the youth experience a particular benefit. Instead of an outcome, my focus was on being present for what was happening and keeping my heart open.

## BEGINNER'S MIND

Although most of us have collected our own set of wounds during our lifetime, some of our clients have experienced difficulties and traumatic events that we can hardly comprehend. There does not appear to be an optimal level of pain that a practitioner needs to experience in order to bear witness to the pain of others, and a practitioner who leads a relatively charmed existence may gain the trust and confidence of clients who have suffered through trauma, loss, and personal despair. On the other extreme, a practitioner who intimately knows suffering may struggle with clients whose lives closely approximate his or her own. Recently, I observed the excellent work of a young man Thomas who, by all intents and purposes, could be characterized as having lived a relatively unscathed life. He is clearly effective with low-income substance-abusing clients, however, because of his compassionate and heartfelt presence, his willingness to deeply accept people for who they are and not judge them, his playfulness, his openness to grow from feedback and from interactions with clients, his self-acceptance including acceptance of his own mistakes and shortcomings, his commitment to meet client needs, his propensity to solicit and utilize client strengths and client-generated solutions, his willingness to take risks, and his beginning-level understanding of counseling theory and interventions.

This practitioner works from what Suzuki Roshi (1970) labeled as beginner's mind, which he once contrasted with the mind of the so-called expert: "In the beginner's mind there are many opportunities, but in the expert's mind there are few" (p. 21).

Expert knowledge does not encumber this practitioner's beginner's mind and the clients reap the benefits of being with a person who goes beyond categorizing them and viewing them simply as addicts. At times, he struggles because of his lack of experience or lack of knowledge regarding substance abuse or 12-step programs; however, he more than compensates for these issues with his openness to learn and to love.

Additionally, this worker manifests characteristics described years ago by Krill (1986) related to vitality, surprise, and playfulness. In addition to his wonderful smile, he tells jokes, lets himself be teased, and projects that being alive is a good thing. It appears as if the large gap of lived experience between him and his clients actually represents an opportunity, similar to how Krill (1986) characterized the preferences of the beat worker:

> He has repeatedly (sought) opportunities to interact and work with people who are most unlike himself . . . . What (he) likes about these clients is the very strangeness, the foreignness of their world

views. For in seeking to understand their unique stances, the worker is forced to move out of his own mindsets and self-images that have become too comfortable and well established. (p. xv)

Thomas celebrates his clients' moment-by-moment lessons as gifts, and I believe that the clients sense that they bring him joy. With an agency structure and various treatment parameters in place, he enters the dance with clients filled with creativity. The guidelines regarding assignments clients need to complete and behaviors and rules with which they need to comply are building blocks or—in Zen language—*forms* for strong back development. These structures provide support for the emergence of the soft front, open-hearted work that reflects the manner in which Thomas bears witness to his clients and their struggles and triumphs.

## WOUNDED HEALER

A fresh view can be valuable—especially if it is combined with the other practitioner characteristics mentioned earlier—however, a wounded healer's perspective may also be a gift for a client struggling with difficulties. The wounded healer, as in the tradition of the shaman, has endured a degree of personal suffering and thus possesses deep wisdom and a willingness to truly see the client in pain. The one who has suffered is able to maintain a strong back presence in the face of client hurt, disappointment, and despair so he or she will not as readily engage in a fight, flight, or freeze response. When a client talks about intense losses, betrayals, disappointments, or fears, the wounded healer is to some degree intimate with how the wounds are experienced in the body, spirit, and mind of the client. If the wounded healer has experienced some success in riding her own waves of despair and pain, she may be a skillful guide for the client. The practitioner who has faced difficult life struggles has familiarity with what it is like to have social, psychological, or biological conditions visit him or her uninvited. The pervasive dark cloud, humiliation, and sense of no escape provide insight into others' experiences. Wounded healers not only have familiarity with the emotional, mental, and spiritual states of clients in pain, they also have ideas about what it takes to move forward. When they speak to clients, they can do so with the impact and force of conviction gained from experience. Clients may be able to feel heard and deeply accepted, especially if they learn that the social worker or counselor has had similar experiences. (We discuss the issue of self-disclosure in a later chapter.)

The wounded healer, however, cannot make assumptions about how much he or she understands the world and the impact of events for her or his client. In other words, we should not assume *to know* what the client is dealing with based on similarity of situations, struggles, or traumas.

Whether we have personally suffered through particular events or not, we may find ourselves gravitating to the most intense aspects of our clients' stories and even fixating our attention in this direction. Stories that are gruesome, traumatic, bizarre, other-worldly, or reminiscent of our own can grab hold of our attention because of how shocking and compelling they are, how voyeuristic we as practitioners are, or how much we are operating with beliefs that client betterment will occur if we dive into the most difficult material first.

## LOOKING INTO THE SUN

Richard Mollica (2006) described the phenomenon of practitioner fixation on the most traumatic elements of the client's story as "looking into the sun." When we look into the sun, we are blinded to the complexities of the person's life as well as to the multiple levels of emotions that the client may experience, including joy. We can easily write our own practitioner story that the client will receive the most benefit through processing the most acute traumatic moments and miss possibilities related to elements that are less graphic and perhaps more immediate.

Mollica (2006) gives an example of how one woman in a Cambodian refugee camp spoke with more pain and expression about how her parents did not let her learn to read and write than about atrocities suffered during the Pol Pot regime in Cambodia. This story was one of many that led Mollica to conclude that a phenomenological approach would best serve traumatized people:

> The basic principle of this method is that a fresh approach to human behavior and relationships can be obtained by the psychologist or doctor by abandoning all currently held theories, opinions, prejudices, and biases. To best help patients, the healing professional has to let go of all of his or her assumptions and "see" what is actually present. It is extremely difficult for practitioners to reject everything they have learned because they've come to depend on conventional labels and diagnostic pigeonholes. (p. 15)

He discusses how this fresh approach, or what we have labeled "beginner's mind," translates to our actual work with traumatized clients:

> Survivors must be allowed to tell their stories in their own way. We must not burden them with theories, interpretations, or opinions,

*especially* if we have little knowledge of their cultural and political background. (p. 60, italics mine)

Bearing witness, thus, involves our capacity, both to clear our minds of preconceived notions and self-constructed stories and to be present for the range of possibilities that the client will present. In the spirit of an ethnographic practitioner (Bein, 2003; Green, 1999), we seek to learn about the client's stories, his or her coping mechanisms, and his or her sense of how life may or may not change for the better. We maintain self-awareness regarding our own propensity to flee or freeze as our own fear or aversion arises, or to fight or become reactive as our anger arises. We do not assume that the most difficult or gruesome events are the most important to focus on. Our minds stay flexible and attuned to cues regarding our clients' needs.

One client, Joanna, who had been labeled as having PTSD brought these lessons home to me. She had suffered greatly in her life through extended episodes of sexual abuse, physical abuse, and domestic violence, the suicide of her mother, the unpredictable appearances and disappearances of her father, the illness and long-term eroding death of the only stable partner she had had in her life, the temporary loss of her children to Child Protective Services, and the mental illness and frightening behavior of her adult child. What I mostly did with Joanna each week was to embrace the totality of her life and love her. She would tell pieces of different stories related to her painful experiences, but I had no agenda regarding how much she needed to cover nor about how deeply she needed to go in her explorations. In accordance with James Hillman's critique on psychotherapy babble—the idea that experiences can be "processed" in the manner that we may process American cheese and place the smooth thin slices in cellophane—I realized that there was no precise formula for healing.

Some meetings involved listening to her stories; sometimes we would make connections between her past survival skills and her present skills, sometimes we would talk about how these experiences precipitated her drug use, sometimes we would talk about how to let go of trying to control her son's life, sometimes we would focus on her forgiving herself for mistakes that she had made (once she was able to face that she did make some mistakes). At the end of our time together, Joanna reflected on how the helping environment allowed her to be honest in a way that she had never been before (she had been in treatment on other occasions). She appreciated my calmness, my caring and self-disclosure regarding some of my own challenges, which I shared despite the agency's general prohibition on this kind of self-disclosure.

## Moving into the Unknown and Responding in the Moment

Most of the time I was with Joanna, I had little idea about what I was doing. The most I "knew" was that each time we would be together for an individual session, it was a special moment in my life. At various times, her anxiety, history of trauma, anger at authority figures, or confusion was disarming. The best I could do was to be with her as well as my own doubts and to help create a sacred space where we would honor each other. I let Joanna see that I did not know the agency's protocol regarding advancements, paperwork, and client assignments—she was my first client at the site. As I fumbled around through the maze of file requirements and requirements for advancement in the program, Joanna fumbled through various parts of her life with me. *Our joint fumbling and stumbling created the story line that we were operating in the unknown together.* Although there were the 12 steps, hastily constructed treatment plan, and program milestones that served as the supposed basis for the direction in counseling, we stayed in the moment—"one day at a time." The lack of control of our client-practitioner interactions ran parallel to the ultimate lack of control that the addict has over her addiction. Awareness of this dynamic helped ground us in the reality that we cannot even promise that we will stay clean and sober tomorrow.

Moment-to-moment decision making regarding what things to say to my client as well as the ways in which to say them reflected a spontaneous process that Schön (1983) characterizes as "reflection-in-action." We may enter relationships with clients with a framework comprised of a theory of change and intervention, notions about "starting where the client is" and an orientation toward empathic relationship-building; however, when the client begins to tell us about her life, we realize that we are faced with moment-to-moment decisions regarding how much to focus versus how much to create space, how directive or passive to be, how self-revealing to be, how confrontative to be, how much to lean forward or how much to sit back, how much to tune into our internal emotional state and/or how much to focus on the session's content, how much to let our compassion flow, or how much to remain poker-faced. Schön (1983) states that our so-called knowing about negotiating these dynamics is tacit, or "implicit in our patterns of action and in our feel for the stuff with which we are dealing. It (in fact) seems right to say that our knowing is *in* our action"

(p. 49). Although our formal professional discourse is currently dominated by so-called evidence-based practice and the language of science, the reality is that often we cannot make definitive and linear statements about our actual, nuanced practice choices and behavior.

Helping practitioners are inevitably artists to some degree. The practitioner-client or worker-community interaction is a canvas that is painted somewhat differently depending on a myriad of conditions. Furman, Langer, and Anderson's (2006) discussion of the poet-practitioner mentions how the poet creates in an environment where "the page is blank and full of both emptiness and possibility" (p. 41). Ironically, though the authors do not mention Zen, *emptiness* is a synonym for boundlessness which, used throughout this book, refers to the essential nonseparateness of beings. As our clients and we dance through space and time together, we create the particular forms we can point to and call "practice."

Furman et al. (2006) encourage us to approach the reality of uncertainty with the "spirit of [a] playful child" (p. 37). This open-hearted creative practitioner is able to truly join and understand the client, to release herself from her own rigidity, and to be vibrant and inspiring. Inevitably, this creative spirit involves us in touching the truth of our client's life and the life that our client and ourselves share moment to moment. Our practice knowledge may assist us in understanding this truth; however, we need to be prepared to set it aside and not become too enamored with its explanatory potential.

As we get back to the story of Joanna, it should be stated that Joanna's own capacity for healing was mobilized, perhaps most significantly through her interactions with fellow seekers in her dual diagnosis group. She went from being a reluctant and angry group member to becoming a teacher, caretaker, and model of courage and effort. She learned how to set limits and how to extend her heart. She shared her life, which included her past and present pain, as well as her triumphs and insights.

Although there was an underlying agency practice framework that helped Joanna thrive, the actual interventions of those who supported her journey through the program could be described as readily as a poet could describe the reasons why she used particular words in a poem. Theory and reductionism may assist in the description; however, the essence of what truly occurred would be missed. Similarly when we try to describe in a linear fashion what *should* happen in therapeutic or helping encounters, we strip down our work in such a bare-bones manner that the profound essence of it is obliterated. Discussions throughout this book are attempts at restoring and giving voice to what really happens when we are with clients.

## BEARING WITNESS AND SOCIAL JUSTICE: THE LARGER WORLD

My practice today was about nondenial.

—Joan Halifax

On the sixtieth anniversary of the bombings of Hiroshima and Nagasaki, an interfaith group organized a series of activities and experiences with the explicit purpose of bearing witness to the entire catastrophe involved in dropping nuclear weapons and killing over 225,000 people, the majority of whom were civilians. (This figure does not include people who died slowly from cancer or other terminal illnesses as a result of the bombings.) How can we make sense of these events so many years later? How are we to connect with what happened and what are we able to do today that reflects something other than feeling overwhelmed and disposed to forgetfulness? What is our responsibility as practitioners often focused on one-to-one helping to bear witness to the larger world's pain?

Throughout a 5-day period, two Japanese survivors of the bombings—one from Nagasaki and one from Hiroshima—told their stories at a peace rally and at other more intimate settings. The survivors, Koji Ueda and Masako Hashida, spoke from their hearts, citing their recollections of the traumatic days in their homelands. Masako Hashida was 15 on August 9, 1945, and shared her vivid memories of grotesquely burned bodies as she ran, first, to a shelter and later to a village some distance away called Nagaura. Not only had she seen melting skin and disfigured bodies and slowly dying victims at the epicenter, she saw suffering at the perimeter village as escaping people tried to heal, sometimes to no avail. Ms. Hashida spoke about how she lived her entire life with a kind of survivor's guilt. She was never sure why she was one of the fortunate ones who had been able to stay alive. Now at 75 years of age, her guilt continued to haunt her.

We all listened to Ms. Hashida with our hearts open. There was infinite patience to go around as her story was clumsily translated by an inexperienced translator. As I entered her world, Ms. Hashida's presence and her story transformed me in an everlasting manner. To this day, partly because of these 60th-anniversary events, I try to align myself with and be guided by principles and practices promoting peace. This intention affects my decisions about where to donate money; how to approach conflicts with colleagues, clients, and family members; and how much to dedicate to social change efforts. I feel gratitude toward Ms. Hashida and for the opportunity to bear witness to the consequences of the nuclear bombings.

Ms. Hashida brought her world of suffering into my heart as a gift, and I was able to hold her pain and learn from her. Her calls for an end to nuclear weapons were especially compelling because she invited us in with her love and sincerity. Although Zen is focused on the present moment, there is an understanding that the present moment contains the past. As we listened to Ms. Hashida and Mr. Ueda, we were struck with how real the events of 60 years ago were. Ms. Hashida's tears and profound grief were in the room with everyone, as were the opportunities for all of us to heal from the tragedy. As Ms. Hashida spoke about her guilt of being able to survive the bombings while many around her had perished, one skilled counselor in attendance lovingly assured her that had she not lived she would not have had the chance to spread her message of peace to the world—what a gift the world would have missed. Ms. Hashida's heartfelt emotional resolution that emerged in response to the counselor's words was quite memorable. Ms. Hashida was not a seasoned and slick speaker; there were no filters separating her from the deepest levels of sincerity and appreciation.

Bearing witness over the 5-day period involved other actions and reflections. Retreat participants became part of a peaceful demonstration at Los Alamos, New Mexico, home of Los Alamos lab where the atom bombs used on Hiroshima and Nagasaki had been developed and manufactured. A march preceding the demonstration provided the opportunity to come face-to-face with a town and its residents who, to this day, are still highly dependent on the presence of the labs. In the tradition of bearing witness, we observed with open hearts all the reactions and responses to our presence, including indifference or apparent indifference. We simultaneously observed our own thoughts, feelings, and narratives as we maintained our silence.

As we marched, I recall a profound sense of acceptance and love for the people who drove by the march and waved in support, the people who had no noticeable reaction, and for the people who, I assumed, tried to disrespect us through their screeching tires and boisterous behavior. I also felt sad that the town's residents were living in a place where the foundation was so embedded in the testing, research, and development of *actual* weapons of mass destruction. Soon I became aware that the Los Alamos residents are not separate from all of us in this country—that we all rest on a culture and a means of production that is directed toward the destruction of human life. Just as there are Los Alamos residents who pretend that the labs do not exist in their town, and as there are Los Alamos lab workers who pretend that they are doing science that is divorced from annihilating human beings, we exist in day-to-day ignorance—with some degree or another of voluntariness—that allows us to deny the reality of our society's priorities.

I remember contemplating the lack of presence of young people during the day of demonstrations. Were their numbers so small because they believed that marches and rallies were ineffective, or were they so preoccupied with what they believed were their personal and private concerns that they preferred not to get involved?

Toward the end of the day, we visited the Los Alamos Lab Museum, operated by the University of California, Berkeley. Some of us were fascinated by the display of weapons and the clinical way that the museum presented the "controversy" related to the social value of nuclear weapons: "Some people think that nuclear weapons create a deterrent for engaging in war, while others say that money invested in nuclear weapon development could be invested in more pro-social causes." I did not want to spend time in the museum, thus I went for a walk and waited outside. I saw a young boy being escorted into the museum by his father, and found myself telling a story about the father's political persuasions—based on his pick-up truck and his son's military style hair cut—and felt sad about our political differences whether they were real or perceived. Other parts of the day involved my trying to stay dry, deciding whether I would go to the local Starbuck's, and wishing that we would get out of Los Alamos.

In the evening, 60 people convened in Santa Fe to process their experiences. Various people made astute observations about what the day meant for them, and their spoken words usually included elements related to their personal likes or dislikes and situations during the day that were either pleasant or unpleasant to deal with. Suddenly, Zen Priest Joan Halifax spoke. She told of how she imagined the human suffering that took place on that day and how her picture incorporated photos and films that she had seen over the years in order to understand—as best as possible—the true devastation on that day. As she described her experience on August 9, 2005, I felt as though she had sat with the suffering people of Hiroshima and Nagasaki in the same manner that she had sat, as a hospice worker, with dying people. She brought her courage and her presence forward to bear witness to the reality of the moment. She had no outcome in mind, and she possessed a sincere commitment to be present for the uncertain terrain. The day's events, the testimonials of our Japanese guests (atom bomb survivors are referred to as *Hibakusha*), her experience with dying people, her work in desperate settings, and her willingness to let go of protective armor and assume the world of other beings all prepared her to bear witness to the reality of an atom bomb attack that took place 60 years ago.

Sixty years ago was today; not only were there survivors in our midst who had direct memories of the events, there was a town, Los Alamos, and a country, the United States, in denial about where the greatest weapons of mass destruction were actually being manufactured, and in denial about who, based on past performance, was the nation most likely to use these weapons.

Thus Joan Halifax recounted the manner in which she was bearing witness to the suffering of the Japanese people that occurred as a result of the U.S. nuclear attack on the country. "Today my practice was about nondenial," she said, and I remembered the profound feeling of gratitude that I had for her as she said those words. Not only had she been willing to so completely face the truth, her process of bearing witness took her beyond our usual preoccupation with what is liked or disliked or what is pleasant or unpleasant.

Much of the time, in our undisciplined mental state, we "hang out" in the space of preferences and likes and dislikes. Recently, in a clinical supervision group, we discussed the dynamics of rating clients as "our favorites" or as the ones "we love" (as implicitly opposed to the ones we do not). While others, including myself, commented on likes and dislikes of the rain, the museum, the various speakers, or going to Starbucks, Joan Halifax commented on the stark experience of connecting with the truth.

Engaging in nondenial blazed a trail of truth and clarity that benefits not only the direct victims of violence or unfortunate acts, such as the *Hibakusha* who visited this country, but also benefits beings who are less directly affected. Joan Halifax's nondenial on this day inspired me to soften my heart and take my seat in the midst of personal and world difficulties. Bearing witness to things as they are is needed medicine for the world. Nondenial is a virtuous, fulfilling, and heartfelt path. As we continue to cultivate a personal and societal field of nondenial, we all experience deeper connections to the truth. Our willingness to face and be present for the painful truth while maintaining strength and an open, soft heart sets the foundation for constructive, loving action designed to relieve suffering.

We bear witness to today's social realities in a similar manner as we do with events that happened 60 years ago. As much as we think we understand the experiences of various communities, it is important that we let go of our treasured ideas and, as best as we can, intimately experience what it means to live the life of others. We nondefensively remain open to the ways that people do not trust us or harbor resentment against us. We love people for their honesty when they let us know how untrustworthy we appear to them as well as for their semi-honesty when they do not want to hurt our feelings. We accept their fears about letting us know how they really feel about us, and we cele-brate their willingness to finally let us into their lives.

We drop our prescriptions for communities about what events should mean to them, how outraged they should be, how they need to understand (in order to be as smart as us) about what the actual social dynamics are, or what risks they should be willing to take to obtain relief or redress for wrongs done to them. Our bearing witness slows us down and moves us away from our scheming, know-it-all mind. It builds trust and heartfelt connection. The solutions and strategies we pursue as we collaboratively endeavor to move forward grow from our deep level of mutual understanding, patience and deep respect, and nonreactivity.

Although the term *bearing witness* had not been used within the structure of Desmond Tutu's theology of *Ubuntu*, the similarities are apparent. Essen-tially, Tutu believed, even the White oppressors championing apartheid were truly sisters and brothers of Black Africans because "they belong to us in the family of God" (Battle, 1997, p. 47). He sought to humanize White South Africans in the eyes of Blacks so that Black South Africans could connect with White people. Tutu offered his manner of thinking and action in the presence of White South Africans:

> What I pick up is the gaze, and in the gaze the presence of a person actively present to me. And the same is simultaneously true of you. The gaze is neither African nor European, but human. (p. 46)

Michael Battle (1997) author of *Reconciliation*, concluded that it was Tutu's spiritual, rather than political, orientation that allowed him to coura-geously and completely face the ravages and devastation of apartheid and in Tutu's words, "stare it down."

# Chapter Seven

# THE MIDDLE WAY: EMBRACING CONTRADICTION AND PARADOX

*Beyond Dualistic Thinking*

> schizophrenia is a garden overgrown
> there are no roads i must travel on
> but i'm finding my way around the thorns
> and making footpaths to ease the journey
> so i know my way again and again and again.

> —Emily Bein

During a clinical supervision session, the familiar words "no big deal" once again came from the lips of a woman I had been supervising over the past 6 months. These words echoed a similar mantra of another 20-something supervisee, who often said, "Things are going okay." Although with both individuals I leaned toward pointing out the limitations of "no big deal" and "things are going okay," these expressed sentiments actually reflected a healthy worldview, and the attitudes behind the words pay dividends for the clients of each of these practitioners. The helper who lives in the world of "things are going okay" or "no big deal" is often prepared not to take personally her client's up and down feelings. As helpers, we are well aware that the people we are trying to assist often do not appreciate our efforts or feel mightily frustrated with their lack of progress. "No big deal" may be part of a laid-back approach that does not react with each sign of client difficulty and is able to ward off the emotionalism of an agency or work setting that is often fraught with change, drama, paperwork pressure, and implicit criticism.

In a talk-radio kind of culture that attempts to create major drama out of, for example, celebrity comments or behavior, "no big deal" or "things are going okay" can represent a breath of fresh air whose source is the wider view, sometimes in Zen called "big mind." While operating in awareness of this wider view, one fully realizes that each moment's occurrences or the self-evaluation of one's performance is quite insignificant when compared to the scale of the universe.

On the other hand, "no big deal" as an ongoing operative principle can lead us to bring an overly laissez-faire approach to our work and our life. As mentioned in an earlier chapter, Mother Teresa is reputed to have said that our actions represent a drop in the ocean, but the ocean would miss this drop were it not there. In other words, "no big deal" may jeopardize our ability to bring a clear intention to our work and our clients. We may lose touch with the power of our smile, or the potential significance of our alert attention and presence. Because our awareness may be slightly dulled, we do not realize the missed opportunities within a client meeting. We thought we were having a good session because there seemed to be some mutual back-patting going on; however, we missed that we could have gone deeper and instead settled with residing in our comfort zone.

Zen practice emphasizes that we embrace the apparent contradiction of "no big deal" *as well as* clear, mindful attention to detail. In bowing, for example, one is to bring her or his intention to the act. We can bow in a half-hearted way, leaning toward the right or the left, and wishing to get the bow over with as soon as possible. Or we can bow in such a manner that at the moment of bowing, there is no thing (nothing) more important in the world. The quality of a bow may seem relatively inconsequential—that is, "no big deal"—and it is. On the scale of what is happening in the world, the manner in which one bows is laughably insignificant.

On the other hand, the way in which we bow or engage in a greeting or other ritual is an opportunity to practice bringing our awareness and intention to the moment. Based on our discussion in Chapter 6 regarding our collective denial, as well as the book's consistent emphasis regarding our need to maintain a conscious presence while with suffering clients, our disciplined—rather than haphazard—bow connects us with possibilities for engaged, alive, and aware interactions. Each moment, in fact, is an opportunity to be alive and present; thus, as we bow, we act as if we are giving our hearts and our concentrated attention to the world. Thus, the manner in which we bow is vitally important—it *is* a big deal.

## BIG DEAL AND NO BIG DEAL EXERCISE

The act of bowing may seem quite foreign and alienating to you—all the better. Engaging in this exercise will be that much more fruitful if that is the case. Imagine a person or situation that is sacred to you. You would like to be present, show your respect, acknowledge your appreciation, or open your heart as you acknowledge this person or place. Bowing is a ritual that brings you to this moment with a clear intention of the moment's significance. As you contemplate bowing, let the swirl of doubts and resistance be part of the process. Tell yourself that you *will not* let yourself go fully—after all, you do have some dignity and why would you do something like this just because the exercise appears in a book.

*Do a "no big deal" bow that incorporates some piece of intention related to respect or acknowledgment but also incorporates your feelings of awkwardness or your thoughts related to how stupid this all is.*

Now prepare yourself to let go of some of the resistance. You are to be mindful of your reluctance and personal discomfort, but your aim here is to bring sincere, focused attention in a manner that truly demonstrates your open-hearted feelings for this person or situation. Fully embracing this ritual means to maintain awareness that nothing is more important in this moment.

*Put your hands together about six inches from your face and do a slow, mindful bow that reflects your open-hearted intention to concentrate your energy into this activity. Let the action cut through your awkwardness or reluctance—you may substitute prayer or candle lighting or some other meaningful ritual.*

In Zen, we embrace the contradiction of how the quality of our actions is both "no big deal" and simultaneously vitally important. We see beyond dualities that depict this kind of issue in the form of a competitive argument and do not attach ourselves to either of the so-called "sides" of the continuum. We live and practice in the Middle Way, where we recognize that the two apparent opposites are actually of the same coin; in other words, completely dependent on one another.

We fill out an intake form with a client, and we realize that we may mechanically run through the form and be just fine. (We are probably not going to be the one to work with this client anyway, and after all, it is important to make sure that all the boxes are filled in.) We also realize that the intake experience is filled with opportunities for the client to feel genuinely heard and for practitioners to be open-hearted and present. We recognize the dangers of "no big deal" when we are doing intakes, and we also recognize the limitations of being wound too tightly and acting as if everything is a "big deal" while we are speaking with our clients.

In fact, we recognize that in each moment, we may simultaneously embrace "no big deal" —which allows space for exploration, creativity— and deep-rooted caring with careful focused attention—which pushes us beyond our comfort zone and communicates the importance of the endeavor.

## DIALECTICAL BEHAVIOR THEORY AND THE MIDDLE WAY

Dialectical behavior therapy (DBT) highlights the apparent contradiction of *change versus acceptance* as one of the major helping dynamics demanding our attention as helpers. The person most responsible for developing DBT is psychologist Marsha Linehan, a dedicated Zen student and aspiring Zen teacher. In working with clients labeled with borderline personality disorder, Linehan (1993) found that cognitive behavioral therapy's "unrelenting focus" on behavior or attitudinal change was invalidating. Consistently communicating that one's ways or thoughts needed to be different did not honor the person, nor did it communicate that the person was worthy of love or worthy of having a life that was worth living. Borrowing from Zen thought, Linehan asserted that radical acceptance of one's life was a vital component—along with change—for one's success. Thus, it became the practitioner's responsibility to not only teach radical acceptance as a skill for clients to learn, but also to embody and exude deep acceptance and validation for clients to be exactly who they were. Because Linehan's methods have been empirically validated through a number of studies (see www.behavioraltech.org for citations), her nondualistic approach has attained additional credibility.

On the surface, radical acceptance appears to contradict change and to reinforce the status quo. On the other hand, change—if singularly pursued — may appear to exclude radical acceptance. A nondualistic perspective, however, allows us to see how each of these elements — radical acceptance and change — interpenetrate one another. Radical acceptance of life as it is (see Chapter 3 for a more complete description), as well as the helper's consistent stance of validation, may lead a client to be able to forgive herself or another, may help her let go of debilitating anger, may allow her to love herself for who she is, or may set the stage for effective action as opposed to residing in denial or paralysis. All of these possibilities would represent significant client change. Greater self-love, as well as an enhanced capacity to see life as it is with some equanimity, represents enormous and profound change for many. Thus, we can see how validation and change are intertwined and interrelated.

On the other hand, coming face-to-face with the reality that change is an inherent part of our lives — we will all get older, many events will happen to us that are out of our control, we will get sick, there will be reasons to celebrate and reasons to mourn, our spiritual life will evolve — assists us in our ability to radically accept the ever-changing world as it is. Change will happen. We can fight this reality or we can accept it and embrace it. Embracing and becoming a full participant in our changing lives enhances our ability to accept ourselves and the world; accepting ourselves and experiencing validation enhances our ability to engage in the changes that will more likely create happiness and well-being. This interpenetration of change and acceptance is applicable whether we are referring to dynamics inherent in individual helping or whether we are involved in family or community efforts.

Embracing the Middle Way means that we first realize that the lines between this apparent duality — validation and change — are not so clear. On a certain level, we may be able to categorize practitioner behaviors that appear more oriented to change and those behaviors more oriented to validation, but ultimately we realize that these distinctions are superficial. Validating a mom who abuses her child and a man who batters his spouse is ultimately about changing them. Working at changing their behavior is ultimately about validating that you believe that they can change in this positive manner and that you wish to be in accord and help them realize their professed goals.

The second implication of the Middle Way for practitioners or helpers is that we do not attach ourselves to either side of the coin. Our resource is the coin and not just the "heads" side or the "tails" side. Seeing the world in terms of these heads and tails is delusional and often is destructive to our helping endeavors.

## COMMON DUALITIES

A monk once asked his teacher Dongshan how to deal with the difficulties that heat and cold pose. Dongshan told the monk that he should avoid them. He said, "When it's cold, cold kills you; when it's hot, heat kills you" (Tanahashi & Schneider, 1994, p. 10).

The universe is to be experienced as it is. When we add ideas such as "this is cold" or "this is hot," our connection to the truth becomes compromised. The raw experience of the moment becomes bracketed with concepts such as cold or hot, good or bad, pleasant or unpleasant, interesting or dull. Our task is to live in the Middle Way, transcending the mind that continually compares, evaluates, and judges. While immersed in our story about the cold, we are not present with what is. We are not intimate with the present moment—the moment where life takes place. Thus, this entire discussion regarding the Middle Way beyond dualities is about transcending concepts, developing clarity regarding the nondualistic nature of phenomena, and not attaching to points of view or to a particular side of the coin.

You may be thoughtful and beginning to ponder whether our discussion about dualities is just another duality. In other words, there are the nondualistic, Middle Way people and the naïve, dualistic people. You are right. We can become attached to nondualism as well. "Look at how good I am at being nondualistic," we may say to ourselves. We realize that ideas presented throughout the book may also be approached as "points of view." We may become attached to becoming accepting over nonaccepting, caring over noncaring, having a strong back and soft front over a weak back and soft front, curious over authoritarian, or present-oriented over thinking ahead. We can even become attached to being nonattached. Ultimately Zen Master Genpo Merzel's words serve as wisdom:

> We are freed from this trap (of paradox) when we realize that there is no way to be free of it. (2003, p. 129)

The remainder of this chapter discusses some of the most common overt or implicit dualities in psychology, social work, or counseling. The medicine for these dualities is Middle Way thought and practice. The manner in which nondualistic thinking transcends the usual discourse within the helping professions cannot be overstated. Practice issues or dilemmas are often—within the dominant Western paradigm—presented as diametrically opposed arguments or controversies. Scholarly debates then proceed regarding the relative value of *DSM*, medical-model mental health practice versus constructivist, strengths-based practice, qualitative research versus quantitative research, micro practice versus macro practice, process-oriented versus outcome-oriented, and practitioner color-blindness versus cultural-sensitivity (although color-blindness is almost always cast as naïve and destructive).

## DISEASE MODEL AND STRENGTHS PERSPECTIVE

This duality is particularly emphasized in social work discourse, where practitioners and scholars bemoan both the increasing utilization of the *DSM* with its simplistic categorization of personal problems and the practice orientations that emerge from a diagnostic system. I join this chorus somewhat when I critique evidence-based practice, so I know the anti-*DSM* side quite well. Basically, the anti-*DSM* people (they usually prefer to be identified as critiquing the disease model) make the following statements regarding the perils of medical model practice:

- People's problems and struggles are complex and occur within context. The *DSM* de-contextualizes people's lives and places them in categorical boxes. The task becomes for helping professionals to develop "intervention technologies" that fit with the symptom-driven categories.
- The use of the *DSM* encourages practitioners to think of solutions in terms of medications or symptom-/behavior-changing interventions rather than empowerment-oriented or context-changing interventions. Thus a child diagnosed with ADD is more likely to receive pills than a plan related to facilitating her or his teacher's effectiveness.
- The use of stigmatizing, disease-oriented labels makes practice conditions ripe for practitioners to see themselves as healthy and their clients as sick. There are philosophical underpinnings regarding the practitioner's role that flow from this healthy versus sick dichotomy; in particular, client opinions about what would be helpful are not taken seriously.
- With prominence given to accurate categorization and analysis of client pathology, the disease model adherent is less disposed to account for and embrace client strengths. Opportunities are missed when clients are not validated for what they are doing well, when their talents are not nourished, and their own skills to reach solutions are not considered or mobilized.

These points are legitimate, and practitioners who pathologize their clients, discount their wisdom or opinions, and reduce and objectify the clients' life essence to their *DSM* label deserve criticism. On the other hand, the diagnostic system itself is not fundamentally flawed, and many suffering people may receive benefit from its utilization. As I reflect about my son's assessment, I remember the sense of validation it brought to my wife and me as parents, as well as to my son himself. We had dealt with a variety of challenges: rage over change in routine, hypersensitivity to sound and texture, nonempathic social interactions, and obsessive narrow interests that brought my son joy but also a degree of anxiety. The label that emerged placed our pain into a container that allowed us to access information, normalize our experience, connect with other parents, talk to teachers, and develop an educational plan that addressed our son's needs. Our son embraced the label, and it helped him transition from merely feeling consistently odd to feeling like he had a place in the world. My daughter's efforts to help her brother were validated as well. He was no longer just a spoiled, in-distress child, he was a child who had a condition that would benefit from her kind efforts.

About 10 years later, my daughter was diagnosed with schizophrenia after a 2- to 3-year period of painful struggle. Although *this* diagnosis did not bring relief, and in fact precipitated intense grief, we gained some clarity about how to proceed. The diagnosis paved the way for the radical acceptance of the pervasive, unrelenting nature of her struggles. She would not necessarily "grow out of" these fundamental challenges, which some "nonpathologizing" therapists had suggested. We would learn to meet each day and appreciate whatever joy or positive interactions arrived. We would bounce around from one psychiatrist with poor listening skills to another, from one medication to another, and through crises, despair, love, confusion, disappointment, and joy. The label *schizophrenia* was a guiding mantra during this time. Keeping this label in our minds organized the process of grinding through the trials and errors of various medications, assisted my daughter in her acceptance of the role medications would have in her life, and provided a vehicle for understanding how her life was unfolding.

Various helpers responded to her as either a schizophrenic or as a unique, precious person who had difficult challenges. It was not the label of schizophrenia that caused people to act one way or another, but the attitudes and meanings attached to the label that determined helpers' dispositions and behavior. Practitioner assertions that they knew what was best, as well as their devaluation of my daughter's experience and wisdom, were the common elements underlying their unskillful actions. It is, perhaps, true that those labeled as mentally ill or drug addicted are susceptible to being treated in a patronizing manner. However, this was not and is not a necessary consequence of the labeling activity itself, but may be an unfortunate outcome.

## THE MIDDLE WAY: BEYOND THE MEDICAL/ DISEASE-STRENGTHS MODEL DUALITY

This discussion shows us the pitfalls and advantages of each side of the coin. Becoming *attached*, however, to either of the two sides destroys our ability to connect with the person in front of us and deal with the nuances, uniqueness, and complexity of her or his situation. Attachment to one side of the coin involves our commitment to a particular ideology; instead, the Zen approach moves toward a direct experiencing of reality through an open, unrestricted lens.

Various New Age or Eastern thinkers had various things to say to my wife or me about the specialness and spiritual nature of hallucinations and the evils of medication. On the other hand, the Research University project people—heavily funded by drug companies and not so good at listening to clients—believed that "their patients" needed to buy the construct that struggles derived from a brain illness required medication for treatment. Both ideological adherents were well-meaning; however, their ideological commitments meant that they were blinded to the actual situation unfolding with my daughter. Instead, they were more invested in their own preconceptions and stories about the way that things are and what people should do.

In the meantime, my daughter's hallucinations were becoming more and more difficult to deal with, creating perils during the day and dramatically disturbing her sleep. Despite these struggles, my daughter was not about to buy the traditional treatment view that one needed to completely dismiss any notion that these visions reflected special insights or connections into other realms or possibilities. My daughter defined the *real issue* regarding the hallucinations as not how "real or unreal" they were, but the fact that they caused her significant distress and made it more challenging to connect with those in the world who were not experiencing them. She did not swallow the mantra that traditional helpers believed was essential for recovery—"this is a disease, so take your medicine." Her decision to take medication came from her own thought process that moved beyond either/or thinking.

When we look at the two apparent sides of the coin, we see how illusory the supposed opposites actually are. As we practice, we commit to not becoming trapped into an alliance with either side and instead see a multitude of possibilities.

## FREEDOM VERSUS STRUCTURE

We offer help in the context of rules and guidelines that guide our own practice as well as our clients' behavior. Structures that grow out of rules and consistent practices may support the helping endeavor through creating safety and a sense of predictability. Our meetings with clients occur at specific times, and there are expectations regarding attendance. As practitioners, we are clear about not engaging in sexual relations with our clients, and our primary aim is to be of assistance to them rather than to view them as meeting our own needs.

For the clients, it may be healthy to surrender to a practitioner's or an agency's rules. Many clients have tried—with numerous failures—to create their own rules or to live haphazardly, as if pleasure was the only guiding principle in their lives. Practice wisdom in substance abuse settings, for example, suggests that strict rules serve to create a healthy container for people who will go astray too easily if left to their own devices.

At first glance, numerous rules and the fairly rigid enforcement of them may appear to be highly oppressive. What about being kind regarding individual circumstances? Isn't it belittling and disrespectful to focus so much on behavior and getting people to conform and comply? Are not people more likely to make longer-lasting changes when they reach decisions on their own about how they will behave rather than succumbing to external demands? We ask these questions from a belief in the duality between structure and freedom.

Interestingly, structure—even very high levels of structure—may ultimately enhance freedom. The process of accepting the structure and no longer fighting against it creates a sense of peace and safety that is quite liberating. When one lets go of his or her reflexive fight-or-flight reactions regarding structure, powerful lessons occur. In fact, a well-developed flight-or-fight reflex may be the oppressive force in the person's life rather than the structure itself.

The presence of structure creates the possibility for the client to actually embrace the structure as it is. As she learns to do this, she also gains practice embracing and surrendering to other apparently oppressive elements of her life. In order to live happier lives, addicts, for example, need to confront the apparently oppressive reality that involvement with drugs needs to cease. In essence, addicts go about structuring their lives in order to experience freedom. They attend programs, they go to 12-step meetings, they work the steps, they stop associating with certain people, they learn how to respond to people who may trigger them, they stop going to certain places, they even stop indulging certain thoughts—all in the name of freedom. Eventually they may translate their lessons regarding structure to other areas of their lives. Committed relationships have explicit rules, such as monogamy, and implicit rules, like doing the best that you can even when things are not working out very well. Jobs also have protocols and expectations regarding time and behavior. Surrendering to the structure of a committed relationship or marriage, as well as to the explicit and implicit demands of the job, can lead to a person's liberation.

Part of radical acceptance is not indulging our always-complaining ego. In Zen, we learn to acknowledge the ego's complaints about how life is not working out the right way. We mindfully witness our disappointment that a cherished image of life has not been realized, and we let go of the story. As we let go of this story regarding how things should have or could have turned out, we return to the present moment of reality. Our return to the present is supported by the understanding that the ego's aim to craft the world in its image leads to greater suffering. We tune into and live in accord with the vibration of the world. As mentioned in the chapter on radical acceptance, we do not adopt the personality of a door mat. Instead, we meet what is in front of us with a strong back and soft heart and proceed skillfully.

The presence of structure teaches us to remain still and not flail about with every change that accompanies the winds of life. This mental stability becomes a precious resource and serves as a foundation for our liberation. Knowing that I need to go to bed no later than 11:30 tonight in order to function well tomorrow, and knowing that I need to treat my wife and my children respectfully tonight provides a container of expectations that can be quite liberating.

Ultimately, we surrender to the reality that our body is not long for the world. We gain a sense of what it is like to be a part of the rhythms that exist in the universe and we desist from viewing ourselves as separate. When we surrender to the structure, we gain a sense of what it is like to surrender to the reality of the larger view.

## FROM CONFLICT TO COLLABORATION: THE MIDDLE WAY AND INTER-AGENCY WORK

The opportunity for polarization and entrenched conflict was palpable at a case conference. I sat down with three women who started off the meeting with some critical things to say about the subject of the meeting—my client. They mentioned how the client was manipulative, not sufficiently motivated, using people to get her way, unnecessarily combative, irresponsible, and possessing a high likelihood of failing. I, on the other hand saw the client as courageous and resilient—she consistently had to battle past demons and trauma as well as her family's notorious reputation in the community. Yes, the client (Terri) was too disorganized sometimes to make it to her various appointments, but the disorganization may have been part of her PTSD. Besides, at 21 she had breast-fed her child for 1 year, had a wonderful bond with her infant daughter, and had enormous success in staying clean and seriously working her program.

The Middle Way between these apparent polarities of view would only occur in an environment of respect. I had to let go of my judgments of the women at the case conference as angry, judgmental recovery types, and I sensed their judgment of me as a co-dependent, wimpy, not street-smart, easily conned-by-a-female male counselor. I made the decision that we all had something to learn from each other, and the meeting proceeded.

I confessed to the practitioners at the case conference that I had not kept adequate account of outside appointments that I knew were important for the client's well-being and her overall success. She was starting to slip in terms of staying accountable, and slipping for her was dangerous. I would have to hold her feet to the fire and be more concrete to assist her to stay on task. I put the case conference participants' story about Terri together with what I had heard about Terri's involvement in group. Her behavior was becoming more erratic. In the name of Terri's being bored or not thinking the group exercises were positive, she was becoming less focused in group. Helping Terri mobilize the part of her that wanted recovery would be important, and having her bring that focus in her moment-to-moment experiences and interactions needed to be discussed.

I had let go of the duality between strengths and problems as well as the duality between support and confrontation. These women were involved with Terri because they wanted to see Terri be successful—that is what all at the case conference had in common. Being supportive (the view that I tend to have of myself) includes confrontation at times. On the other hand, in order to confront, you must support the person and her growth. My tone in the meeting was not about them versus me or them versus us (me and the client). I made some points about Terri and my perceptions of her that the other practitioners were able to hear.

First, I asked the question about how hard it would be to work with Terri, when—as they said—so many other young people are not successful. I did not sneak in an underhanded accusation about one of the counselor's negativity; the inquiry was from a stance of curiosity and not-knowing. If I had seen so many young people struggle, I may have said the same thing. The worker clarified that these thoughts cross her mind, but that she manages to stay positive when she is working with everyone.

I had the wish that they consider that my client's behavior was not necessarily from negative intentions. I reviewed history that they already knew about her and discussed how some of her behavior reflected all that she had ever seen. I added that with her own history of abuse, the loss of her boyfriend to prison, and the constant unpredictable and volatile behavior of her mom, Terri tries to do what she can in order to survive a life that seems chaotic. She had already lost a child to Child Protective Service as a teen; she will try to get her way so as to keep the ground steady under her feet. As I saw the heads in the room nodding, I added, "and you know that word—*manipulation*—I really have a hard time with it because it implies shameful behavior and perhaps some negative intention on behalf of the manipulator. I think most of the time Terri is just trying to survive."

Somehow we had come together as a foursome to the degree that a few minutes later, one of the women stopped herself from saying "manipulation." I pointed out how wonderful it was to see her purse her lips to make the *mm* sound and then open her mouth to allow another word to come out. We all affectionately laughed about the effort.

The Middle Way for working with this client was established with the realization that we were all interested in her best interests. We dropped our stylized way of doing things and considered inputs about how to most be effective. We let go of our attachments to one side or the other of the confrontation versus support duality as well as the strengths versus problems duality. This meeting was integral to this client's continuance in the program. Had we stayed stuck in our initial "camps," or views, the meeting had the ingredients for a disaster. We were able to transcend our treasured notions and ways of looking at things and were able to embrace multiple perspectives without becoming attached to a side of the polarity.

## SYSTEM CHANGE: SURRENDER TO THE BOX/BE OUT OF THE BOX

Our agency's or work site's rules, norms, and regulations can sometimes feel stifling. Sometimes external forces like insurance companies define the help that we may provide. Other times, our agency or institutional practices are rigidly prescribed, so that it looks like *their* structural needs are being addressed at the expense of clients' needs and best interests. Additional structural demands are heaped on us, such as paperwork and meetings. Although we commonly speak about "compassion fatigue," practitioner burnout often occurs because of structural issues and concomitant lack of support occurring at human service settings.

Surrendering to the box represents a radical acceptance strategy. There are often site-based elements that constrain our ability to help another and that transcend or compound either the client's ecological or personal difficulties or the practitioner-client relationship challenges. At our sites, there are people we can serve and people we cannot serve; there are time limits regarding service; there are things we can do and things we cannot do; there are practitioners within the setting that clients may see and people within the setting—because of assignments or caseload—that they cannot meet with. Many times, we are not supposed to give people rides, money, gifts, or even an additional session. Our clients are not supposed to get too unruly, rude, ungrateful, or—my favorite terms—"inappropriate" or "manipulative."

Surrendering to the box means making peace regarding these various constraints. If we rail against the very places that serve as vehicles for helping—however limited and flawed we believe them to be—we are setting ourselves up for frustration and ineffectiveness. We recognize that we have signed on for offering help within this setting, and we do the best we can to embrace the limitations and be there for our clients. Additionally, we stay on top of our paperwork and avoid making these less-enjoyable tasks so odious that personal procrastination and internal mental warfare overtake us and render us useless.

Surrendering to the box does not mean we are apathetic, docile sheep who never question or resist oppressive or dysfunctional practices. However, our ability to accept and not demonize the institutional structure we operate within allows us to develop clarity about what needs to change, as well as to initiate constructive strategies to make this change happen. Our equanimity serves as an example for our clients, establishes credibility vis-à-vis system players that we are targeting for change, and protects us from becoming unbalanced, angry, burned-out, and ineffective. We approach change efforts with a soft front that includes our focus on maintaining compassion and respect (process focus). Additionally, our strong back is needed to take risks and pursue outcomes despite encountering organizational resistance.

## CASE EXAMPLE: IN THE BOX/OUT OF THE BOX

During group supervision, a practitioner discussed a teen-age boy who was requesting service. The practitioner had seen this boy for an intake session as well as one individual session and felt a connection with him. Apparently the boy also felt a connection because, although he "disappeared" from the agency for a month, he wanted—at the time of the clinical supervision session—to meet with the same practitioner. The boy appeared to be quite fragile—he was having hallucinations, receiving very little support from home, and had attempted suicide. The agency was generous about seeing the youth and was even willing to have the practitioner meet with him at a satellite location (much beyond the accommodations that would be made at many sites I have been familiar with). Despite the agency's generosity in this regard, there was the matter of who would do the new intake for the boy. It seemed that the practitioner who would eventually provide counseling for the youth was not supposed to do these kinds of intakes because he was not officially part of the program that the boy was to be enrolled in.

The dilemma about who would conduct the intake arose because the boy said that he wanted to see only one particular individual at the Center. After all, he had been suffering hallucinations, had just tried to kill himself, and felt embarrassed about all he had gone through. At that moment, the standard responses ensued in the supervision room regarding the boy's insistence. Statements such as "this is the only way we can run this program . . . he has to come in through the established intake channels," and "he can't call the shots, that's giving him too much power" were both mentioned. The group participant who was most insisting on the standard intake procedure was part of agency administration and higher than me in the organizational hierarchy.

Before I discuss my intervention, I need to say that I had practiced at this site with enormous respect for the work and efforts of all the people involved and I had surrendered to the box. The surrendering meant that I did not pretend to know what was best, that I consistently embraced a learner role (even though I was called the clinical supervisor), and that I was not reactive when situations would arise that I had questions or doubts about.

Before I spoke to the supervision group members about the case content, I addressed what I perceived to be the needs of the people attending the supervision group. I announced that my questions would be provocative in order to prepare the practitioners in the room. They were used to my provocative questions and they came to trust that I asked them in a spirit of love, respect, and playfulness. My ability to advocate stood in contrast to my performance at prior work settings. When I raised controversial issues in these situations, my questions or comments were often laced with a sense of moral superiority and righteousness, my seething and leaking anger, and ultimately, my despair sprouting from an internal belief that I would probably have no effect on the outcome.

(Continued)

I invited the group to tune in to the plight of the young boy, and I asked the participants how they would feel if the child refused to come to the intake as we had designed it, never enrolled in our program, and then killed himself a short time later. If we could see this scenario unfold in the crystal ball, would we do the same thing? There was not a trace of anger or self-righteousness in my voice. I ultimately radically accepted what people were doing, and fortunately at this particular site, I profoundly trusted the intentions of all involved. As the discussion evolved, creative problem solving occurred that involved giving the young man various opportunities to make decisions, and all agreed it would be a good idea to allow his preferred counselor to *accompany* him to the intake session.

Because I had surrendered to the box—the structure of the agency, the way it worked and the way decisions were made—I was able to step outside of the box and ask the agency to go along with me. Embracing the box and stepping outside the box become quite different than the fight-or-flight responses that I have practiced in my career, which tend to be ineffective and lead to frustration. When we embrace the box or the structure, we are not selling out, *and* when we step out of the box and risk, innovate, or rebel, we are not being reactive, angry, and despairing children. We learn that in order to step out of the box, we need to be in it. We learn, as well, that in order to be truly alive in the box, we need to have the capacity to step outside.

## DUALITIES GALORE

In the chapter on bearing witness, we explored the duality of boundaries and boundlessness. We occupy the Middle Way between one apparent perspective that recognizes that pain belongs to no *one*, thus it is held in the boundless client-practitioner space, and the other view that posits that our healthy boundaries allow us to not become awash with everyone's difficulties. The discussion on boundaries suggests that they are healthy for our clients and ourselves. Ultimately, we live as if there are boundaries in a fundamentally boundless world and we recognize that it would be folly to embrace only one side of the coin. There are other dualities that are important for us to deconstruct. I would love to hear from as you explore them in your practice or in writings:

- Joviality versus seriousness
- Color blindness (universal concepts) versus cultural (emic) awareness

- Protecting self versus risk/growth
- Support versus confrontation
- Involvement versus detachment
- Individual responsibility versus collective responsibility
- Qualitative versus quantitative
- Direct versus nondirect
- Micro versus macro
- Hierarchical versus democratic
- Goal oriented versus process oriented
- Advocacy versus collaboration
- Independence versus dependence or interdependence
- Expert-driven versus postmodern
- Agency/practitioner agenda versus no agenda
- Knowing/known versus unknowing/unknown
- Reality versus possibility
- Creating dialog versus being instructive and pushing
- Letting go versus demanding or fighting for change
- Body versus mind
- Teacher versus learner
- External motivation (praise/rewards/consequences) versus internal motivation
- Spiritual versus material
- Spontaneous versus deliberate
- Conceptual versus nonconceptual
- Expectations versus no expectations

As you looked through the list, perhaps you began to experience some freedom realizing that no part of the apparent duality needs to be defeated or excluded. We in fact embrace them all and sense the interdependence of these concepts.

A final example brings home the nondual nature of existence. Throughout the book, we have discussed the Zen perspective on how concepts add layers of evaluation and comparison that interfere with the actual and direct experience itself. We have been encouraged to let go of our wishes to create certainty and instead embrace uncertainty and adopt an open-hearted approach with our clients. It has been said that this approach enhances our ability to be present. Ironically, this path of practice is laced with concepts. The very suggestion that our work as helpers is fundamentally about *uncertainty* is, in fact, a concept about our work. Strong back/soft front, caring, curiosity, radical acceptance, bearing witness, and nonduality are concepts as well. In order to speak about a nonconceptual approach with our clients, we become conceptual. Just as with the dualities listed above, we realize that we are best able to respond to the realities of people in need when we are able to embrace the Middle Way between conceptual and nonconceptual. We flow back and forth from side to side, realizing that the "sides" depend on one another and realizing that it makes little sense to attach ourselves to one point of view.

# Chapter Eight

# HAVING THE CONVERSATION: MAKING SPACE FOR CLIENT SPIRITUALITY

*Beyond the Great Taboo*

We understand the benefits of taking our seat with clients while embodying a strong back and soft front. We sit down in the midst of uncertainty and difficulty and we focus on maintaining a mindful presence and an open compassionate heart. We live in the awareness that each moment is sacred and we do our best to reflect the importance of each action. Judgments, distractions, and inclinations to run or rebel all visit, and we learn ways to observe them and let them go. We are aware that clients deeply attend to whether we care, and we do not want our own temporary feeling states, thoughts, or judgments to get in our way. Our breath brings us back to curiosity and radical acceptance; we consistently find inspiration from our clients' lives of heroism and resilience. Our sense of spaciousness allows us to hold what some may consider as contradictions or dualities. Our clients may have a diagnosis and yet transcend that diagnosis; we ourselves play with these apparent dualities realizing our interconnection and boundlessness on the one hand, and the need for boundaries on the other.

This description summarizes the spiritual story found in the first seven chapters of the book. As we grapple with how the book's practices and ideas fit with our own religious orientation and spiritual or nonspiritual background, each of us weaves a story about how to apply these lessons. Despite our diversity regarding how we apply the book's principles in the field, we sense that mindful and open-hearted practice leads to enhanced self-care and personal wholeness as well as enhanced effectiveness with clients. True to the Zen tradition, we do not keep the goodies for ourselves and we allow the client's spirituality to enter the room.

There are many reasons why client spirituality seems like a taboo topic. First, we have been taught that answers to our clients' problems reside in the social and biological sciences. We must therefore toil within these arenas to understand our clients' lives and find the most useful interventions or solutions. Engaging in the dialogue around spirituality threatens the helping profession's domain of expertise regarding the client's dealings and threatens our hold on specialized knowledge about how to help. Are we really prepared to hear just how much our client says she benefits from prayer? How curious and mindfully nonjudgmental are we as our clients discuss how God is testing them; how things in their life "happen for a reason," or how they wished that God would not punish them so much? How much do we recognize that client spirituality holds the potential for client betterment and positive outcomes and how willing are we to delve into this area even if it has not "come up" during our sessions?

Second, we imagine that if our client starts quoting from the Bible or Quran we will feel lost or inadequate. Various students have told me that they may feel somewhat competent helping a person with a similar religious background, but they are doubtful about helping people who have a different religious or spiritual orientation.

Third, we are unsure of our service site's view regarding spiritual or religious matters. When we work at a substance abuse agency, we are clear that their 12-step orientation promotes the discussion of spiritual matters. When we work at public agencies such as Child Protective Services or settings that contract with the state or county, we are less confident about bringing up issues of religion or spirituality with our clients.

Fourth, we do not trust ourselves with carrying on this conversation in a way that is respectful and maximizes client self-determination. Some of us have an anti-religious or anti-spiritual bias (Hodge, 2005). On the other hand, there are practitioners who have such strong convictions or belief systems that they are concerned that they will overwhelm their clients and be tempted to engage in some form of proselytizing. Various Christian practitioners particularly reported this thoughtful concern.

Fifth, we are not confident about the relevance of this conversation for particular issues and specific populations. Some practitioners and students believe that teens will not be interested in spiritual or religious matters, for example. Others are cautious about engaging in spiritual discussions with schizophrenics because of the commonly held belief that such exchanges could enhance their delusional system. Some are concerned that if they were to engage with a gay client, for example, who feels depressed because of his church's viewpoint on homosexuality, they will not be adequately prepared to engage in a dialog around issues such as specific biblical scripture.

## MOVING BEYOND OUR FEARS AND CONCERNS

We need to realize—as Hodge (2005) argues—that religion and spirituality may be a liberating and health promoting force in the lives of our clients and not examining its interface in our clients' lives is often irresponsible. Since our purpose is to help, we need to understand what help means to our clients and the packages they believe that help comes in. We enter the uncertainty of this inquiry and attempt to understand how the client's bigger picture, spiritual view, or her or his particular religious practices make a difference.

It makes little sense to say that we will inquire about spirituality but we will not talk about religion. The dualism between religion and spirituality is artificial when it comes to the world of our clients. We may find out that our client (we will call him Walter) has dealt with trauma all his life through believing that God has had a purpose for him. We may learn that music gives him the opportunity to touch the divine and provides him sanctuary, and that he has forgiven the perpetrator of the violence that he has suffered. We have done well understanding elements of Walter's spiritual life and how his spiritual views contribute to his resilience and strength. Asking religiously oriented questions does not push the envelope unnecessarily.

We may want to learn whether Walter goes to church or experiences any kind of social support regarding his spirituality. Religion is the *form* that spirituality often takes. It comes in packages of particular belief systems with names such as Catholic, Muslim, Jewish, Christian, or Buddhist and there are places of worship that religiously oriented people sometimes frequent. People also trace their religion back through their ancestors. Obviously, people have all kinds of combinations regarding the manifestations of their religious and spiritual lives. Some people start with the formality of religion and become more spiritual over time. Some people start with some religious training, leave their place of worship to develop their own sense of spirituality, then return to a place of worship to gain community and structure. The nuanced stories are numberless, and interestingly, by and large, *people appreciate telling them.*

We mindfully watch our fears and concerns rise and fall and we let our curiosity flourish. Our clients sense that we care because we risk venturing into an area of intimacy that others have avoided. We radically accept our clients' story about their spirituality and religion. Because the spiritual stories are so profound, clients may experience benefits that transcend the mere enhancement of the practitioner-client working relationship. One acquaintance reported to me the benefits that he received through one of my student's focused questions regarding his spirituality. Through "having the conversation," he became increasingly conscious that he had let his spiritual and religious life lay dormant for too long. While he and the interviewer were "having the conversation," he became aware of the preciousness that his spiritual and religious life made available for him. He had been living a life — for too long — of distraction and needed to return to the essence. The interviewee reported that this discussion helped him renew his focus on religious practices and it helped him drop the depression that he had suffered during the year leading up to the interview. It is important to note that the interviewer was Jewish and the interviewee Catholic.

We create space to have the conversation because we know of the transformational impacts that religious activity or spiritual thought and practice may have. We do not have to be religious scholars any more than we have to be medical experts to talk about someone's struggle with a particular disease. Our strong back creates a container in the midst of not knowing. Often, just learning what religious practices or spiritual beliefs mean to the client is enough. Other times, we may share our limited — or more-than-limited — understanding of their beliefs. Other times, it may make sense to consult with pastors, priests, rabbis, or the literature to learn more.

Our soft front opens to the stories that our clients discuss with us. Sometimes these stories are embedded with ambivalence, pain, conviction, liberation, support, apathy, faith, confusion, or peace. We are present for whatever arises and accept that it is our client's narrative.

We notice that because we are open to having the conversation the conversation arises much more frequently than before. We actually hear instead of ignore clients when they make references such as: "I hope that God helps me through this," or "Maybe I should go home tonight and pray." We follow up with our curious mind and open heart and attempt to learn more.

## AGENCY CONTEXT AND RISK

We soon realize that these conversations are not a sidebar to being a helping practitioner, nor are they to be reserved for hospice clients or clients at faith-based organizations. Spiritual life is too important to be left out of the equation, and we realize that, ethically, we must make an attempt to understand its role in our clients' lives. We acknowledge the spiritual and religious involvement that our clients have and we may ask them questions so that they can reflect on whether this source of strength is being tapped the way that they would like. We also make space for clients who do not profess any religious affiliation or who state that they do not consider themselves to be "spiritual." To borrow a phrase from Duncan, Miller, and Sparks (2004), spirituality might not be a part of some clients' "theory of change."

Because we are confident and less fearful about having the conversation, we do not go looking for site or agency policy that either affirms or denies whether to address this topic. Whether we are in a county agency or a public school, we put our client's well-being at the center of our agenda and seek to understand his or her vehicles for achieving success. The groups of people we had assumed would not care about the conversation surprise us with how profound religion or spirituality has been to their story of resilience. I have worked with gang members, for example, who have a strong spiritual base and engaged in particular religious practices; however, they have little opportunity to explore that part of their lives with helpers. Similarly, we do not make stereotypical assumptions about schizophrenic clients. At times, the discussion of God needs to be brought to focus; however, many clients are coping with their struggles through spiritual or religious beliefs. Some pray or chant every time hallucinations become intense or voices intrude with punishing messages. Don't we want to know about these experiences? (See Tenowich, 2007, http://newsinitiative.org/story/2007/07/24/schizophrenia_talking_to_god/ for a compelling individual story and the needs and dilemmas of having the conversation with a schizophrenic man.)

Our agenda is not to have clients buy into our particular brand of religion or spirituality. As we discuss cases with our supervisors or program directors, we take the risk that this kind of work—on behalf of clients—is appreciated and understood. We cite the increasing literature (Canda, Nakashima, & Furman, 2004; Gilbert, 2000; Hodge, 2005; Murphy & Dillon, 2008) that states that working from this perspective is responsible and ethical, and we listen—with a strong back and soft front—to our agency administrators' arising fears and discomfort (if these should occur). We bear witness to whatever agency resistance may be present and we respond in a response-able manner.

## ETHICAL ISSUES

Having the conversation does present potential ethical dilemmas. Many of us are attached to a particular path of salvation or have some clear ideas about what religious practices should be followed in order to improve our life and get closer to God. As helping practitioners, we do what we can to let go of our own frameworks and to see them for what they are—our stories about ultimate truth or about what it takes to achieve everlasting peace. We commit to working within the client's frameworks to honor the client's cultural map and her or his self-determination.

---

### CONTEMPLATION EXERCISE

"Having the conversation" demands rigorous honesty and self-awareness. Take some deep breaths and let yourself imagine sitting down with a client and addressing issues related to spirituality/religion. Contemplate these questions: What are my intentions? How much am I willing to let the client lead the way and how much are my own perspectives creeping in? To what degree do I create space for my clients to *not know* about their religious or spiritual orientation, to be antireligious, to be confused about the role that religion or spirituality plays in their life, or to hold beliefs and engage in practices that seem exotic and unfamiliar?

---

Unfortunately, our human insecurities, comparing minds, judgmentalism, and narcissism find room for expression in religious life. Our insecurity manifests in the form of fearing difference. Many of us derive comfort when the size of "my group" grows larger and there are fewer "others" walking around with ideas and perspectives that are different. Our comparing and judgmental mind manifests through our keeping score about which religious orientation is *the best*. The followers of the religion with the lowest score are branded, sometimes, as a collection of lost, misguided puppies. The liberating nature of some of our individual religious experiences as well as the insular character of religious practice creates the conditions for this kind of thinking. We are not bad people for making comparisons and having judgments; our task is to be aware that we sometimes have stories about whose religion is better. We notice the stories for what they are—stories—and we make the commitment to not become attached to them.

Finally our narcissism creates blind spots regarding the value and benefit of others' perspectives and practices. We know *the truth*, essentially because we believe it to be true or because people whom we trust have told us that it is true, or because we have had personal experiences that seem to confirm that it is true. We may feel narcissistically injured or rejected when someone chooses a different path, which may include the choice of no path at all. We insist to ourselves that we *know* the way, and we have trouble coming to grips with someone who in effect says: "Your way does not work for me," or "I am not willing to try your way."

It is difficult to maintain the relative perspective of the truth, when, as a person of faith, you deeply believe that you touch the truth. The following dialogue is an approximation of what has occurred numerous times between devout believers and me:

**Devout Believer:** I feel like this is not just about my *belief* about truth, what I believe *is* true.

**Bein:** My idea is that you have a story about the truth and part of that story involves that you know what the truth is and others do not. I sense, though, that you don't like my use of the term *story* because it treats your version of the truth as a relative experience rather than as the absolute truth.

**Devout Believer:** You're right. I don't like how you use the term *story* to describe my faith. My faith is more than a story.

**Bein:** I am sorry about that—that is the best language I can come up with to address the phenomenon of emotionally charged people coming into conflict with one another, each believing that his or her tradition or belief system is *the* right one. The language that I use becomes my own story about how we can respect each other's beliefs. I don't use the word *story* to be demeaning but to remind us how each of our versions are different *and* acceptable. (Acceptable here means that they are able to be accepted, not that they meet some particular standard of worthiness.)

**Devout Believer:** I understand that.

Of course, this is my story about what happens in our interactions. I get to make the insightful comments in my story. There are other stories about what happens in these kinds of interactions.

## FINGERS POINTING TO THE MOON

This famous Zen metaphor has usefulness here. In Zen, the moon is often a symbol of enlightenment. It is the state that we wish to arrive at. There are many stories about what the journey looks like and many descriptions about what enlightenment is. All of these depictions are words or concepts that point to the moon. They are not the moon itself. We often mistake the fingers for the moon. We believe that if we adopt one of the fingers then we have arrived.

This metaphor may be useful in understanding the phenomenon of religion and other life paths. Many of our human goals (and these goals as manifested in the teachings of the world's religions) are similar. We seek to understand or touch a sense of the divine or that which is greater than our small, worried self. We seek to cultivate compassion and an ability to live and get along with others. We wish to see the sacredness or specialness in the smallest acts and beings. We try to understand our place in the world and experience an abiding, universal love that is our refuge. We try to gain some peace about where we came from and where we are going when our body perishes. The moon is the realization of the above: loving and appreciating life, getting along and being compassionate with others, being at peace with dying, and feeling a sense of belonging and purpose. There are many fingers that point to the moon. We spend a lot of time on this planet arguing and fighting about which finger is better. We mistake the finger for the moon itself. In the Zen story, the finger is not important. That we live a life of integrity, joy, generosity, appreciation, sacredness, and peace is of concern. We all take different paths to get there.

## FOUNDATION OF RESPECT

We establish the deepest level of respect for each other's perspectives in order to have the conversation. We do the best we can to drop our own story about how right we are, and we engage our curious mind as we listen to our clients. In a classroom setting, we acknowledge that some of our differences may be hurtful or difficult to bear. We make clear that our intentions are not to hurt and often decide that the sincere exploration of these issues is worth it. I have found that framing particular beliefs as stories has helped gay students feel protected from being condemned by a "knower of absolute truth," and it has given some Christian students the opportunity to explore their own beliefs rather than staying underground with them. Fruitful dialog and actual friendship has emerged from these opportunities.

With clients, we understand that each person's path will be different. We do not have to be an expert about each of the fingers, but we may explore the moon and a finger or two with our clients. Sometimes we develop a sense that a greater level of dedication or discipline applied to a particular finger has the potential to make a difference for a client. We sense that meditation may help an anxious client or consistent prayer may benefit someone who is deeply depressed. We respectfully discuss whether either of these methods has ever been part of the client's repertoire and, if not, had he or she ever considered either of them. We move slowly and respectfully and ask if this area of exploration is okay. We may have simple ideas to offer regarding prayer or meditation if our client requests them or we may have thoughts about whom to refer the client to. In the end, just as we do regarding other areas of the client's life, we respect client self-determination and do not get attached to whether he or she follow through with any of the fingers.

## ALTERNATIVE STORIES

When Bobby Griffith was about 5 years old, he already felt different than a lot of other boys. He enjoyed playing with dolls and did not seem to fit in easily with his male peers. As he reached adolescence, it became apparent that Bobby was gay. He certainly did not choose this "lifestyle." Bobby wanted to please his parents, and it was obvious that—with his parents' Christian fundamentalist beliefs—they would have a difficult time accepting him and his sexuality. Additionally, Bobby believed in God and the teachings of the church. He felt that he was letting God down and that he was fundamentally flawed and sinful. He went to counseling to stop being gay and on the intake form under reason for visit "he wrote that he wanted to be the kind of person God wanted him to be" (Miller, 1992, p. 83). After failed attempts at conversion counseling (attempting to convert Bobby to becoming heterosexual), Bobby attempted to piece his life together. Unfortunately, Bobby believed that he could no longer turn to God for comfort because he believed that God no longer accepted him. His wonderful relationship with his mother was fractured because his mother could not come to terms with Bobby's emerging sexuality. "Every effort to affirm his homosexuality was met by (his mother's) resistance and quotations from the Bible" (p. 84). Bobby's father drifted out of the picture.

Bobby's pain, self-hatred, isolation, and rejection led him to commit suicide 2 months after his twentieth birthday. His mother, Mary, began a quest for meaning immediately after his death. "Was her son innocent and with God in Heaven? Or had Bobby's name been erased from the Book of Life as promised to the sinful in Revelation?" (Miller, 1992, p. 85). She continued to search for answers to these questions within spiritual and religious circles. She eventually sought an alternative story for all that had occurred. Her quest was courageous. She allowed for the possibility that there was another religious narrative that would displace the one that she had held onto so tightly. As a result, of her work, "Mary . . . squared her religious faith with her own sense of love for her son. She (became) convinced that Bobby was the kind of person that God wanted him to be" (p. 86). Mary Griffith eventually became a national figure and speaker for Parents and Friends of Lesbians and Gays (PFLAG).

We will meet other Bobby and Mary Griffiths. Of course their stories will not be identical, but some serious patterns and similarities may be present. Our fears and doubts about addressing religion and spirituality may arise, and we likely will be able to fall back on some good reasons for not moving forward. Many of us know little about scripture; how could we keep up with Mary in a religious discussion? We may not be sure how our service site would feel about our engaging Mary in this kind of conversation. How can we have the conversation and respect Mary and *her* pain? Maybe, we tell ourselves, that because the whole affair is so sticky we would be better off avoiding it.

We enter the conversation with our strong back and soft front. We are, perhaps, not an expert on Mary's religion, and because of our limited knowledge and the other contextual issues, we enter into the unknown. We bear witness to two people in pain, and we tell the story of Bobby Griffith. It is a story of hope and failure and new possibilities. Rachel Naomi Remen, MD (2007), has said "nothing has the power to change the world like a story can." Perhaps our courage to tell the Bobby Griffith story will save someone's life.

# Chapter Nine

# DEALING WITH FAILURE

*Beyond Cognitive Solutions and the Paradigm of Blame*

*The only safety lies in letting it all in—*
*The wild with the weak; fear,*
*fantasies, failures and success.*
*When loss rips off the doors of*
*the heart, or sadness veils your*
*vision with despair, practice*
*becomes simply bearing the truth.*
*In the choice to let go of your*
*known way of being, the whole*
*world is revealed to your new eyes.*

—Danna Faulds

The audience was boisterous and seemed to be increasingly dissatisfied. One or two people starting confronting each of the Zen teachers that evening, and the teachers and the attendees appeared stuck in a back-and-forth process that yielded little fruit. I had always seen Joan Halifax, one of the two speakers, command the audience with her deep wisdom, poetic language, profound presence, connection with her listeners, and delightful humor. Today she appeared to be helpless and ineffective with this particular group. She had been battling pneumonia on the trip, was unfamiliar with the culture of the setting, and the hostility of some of the participants appeared to catch her off guard. The following day at breakfast, I wanted to hear her impressions of what went on the night before. The following is an approximation of what she said:

> "There I was sitting there," she said. "Watching the intense crowd and frustrated faces. Realizing that the evening was deteriorating and that I did not have the strength to do much about it nor the knowledge of what to do. I started to take it all in and then *I just settled into the reality that this is a complete failure.*"

Hearing those words come from the mouth of my esteemed teacher was so liberating. We usually do all we can to run from the f-word. We work so hard at achieving success or at appearing as if we have it all together. When we do slide and have difficulties, we feel deeply ashamed. Our major strategies then become either to hide the failures as best as we can from ourselves and others and/or to explain away failure so that no one will think it is our fault.

The following discussion of failure is not about claiming how events are, in fact our fault or not our fault, nor is it about how to lay blame on the door-step of those who have failed. Instead we learn to feel at peace with the idea that we have failed—in the sense that we have been part of an overall experience of failure.

As a parent, I have dedicated my efforts at helping my children have a happy and fulfilled life. The ultimate failure for a parent is when his or her child is in a major state of distress or crisis. Of course, I may be able to point to contributing elements to my child's distress that were out of my control (e.g., biological issues, abusive peers), and I may arrive at fair descriptions and explanations for why I was not as effective as I could have been (e.g., ignorance, fear, my father's weak back was a poor model for dealing with crisis). When I dwell in this cognitive world of explanations and contributing factors, however, I do not experience the same level of peace as when I accept the reality that I failed.

This discussion perhaps causes pain and discomfort for some of you. You have worked hard to realize that growing up with abusive parents or living in a violent relationship is not your fault. You have learned to shed self-blame and shame for events and circumstances that you had no control over. You may think that to embrace failure is to buy into the package of blameworthi-ness and shame. Instead, I ask you to consider the universal nature of failure. Many of us have had failures in our family lives, many of us have had mar-riages or partnerships that have failed, all of us fail with our clients repeat-edly. The notion here is to embrace failure in such a way that we *do not* suffer the shame that comes with events, even traumatic ones, that visit our lives and, ultimately, as discussed in Chapter 6, deliver us into the world of personal humiliation. Failure is a universal experience from which no one is immune. We accept that we will all receive our own heavy dose of failure and when it comes our way we realize that we are connected with the human experience, and, in particular, our clients.

## EMBRACING FAILURE AND CONNECTING WITH CLIENTS

As we become more comfortable with our own failures, clients experience that they do not have to hide from their failures. As mentioned throughout this book, our relationships with clients are not reflections of dualities — in this case between those who have failed (the clients) and those who have not failed (the practitioners). We all live through catastrophes and troubles and, at times, we all feel like failures. Facing our own mistakes as well as our stories of failure may help us feel liberated. We radically accept that we and failure have joined together, and we reach a level of peace about failure in our lives that does not necessarily occur when we cognitively dissect or reinterpret situations.

Some life events or circumstances are such that there is little opportunity for reframing or other cognitive-focused interventions (e.g., pointing out distortions in thinking) to provide relief. In one case, a young woman (Luisa) is heroically raising an infant despite constant reminders of how she lost her first child when she was 16 years old. As a 16-year-old mother, she essentially chose methamphetamines and the life of the streets over caring for her son. This smart young woman knows about the addictive process. She was able to rationalize that "it was the drugs talking" and "it was addiction" that took control of her life and made her do things that others addicts do. She was also aware that between her stepfather's sexual advances and her mother's addiction, notorious temper, and nonprotection, she received little modeling about how to be a mother. At the time of her son's removal, she knew that her son was better off being raised by others; thus Luisa's "letting go" of her son could be recast as a heroic act. Her son serves as Luisa's constant inspiration for taking care of her 10-month-old daughter. Again there is opportunity to revisit the narrative of losing her son as paving the way for being a wonderful parent for her daughter.

There is abundant cognitive material here for Luisa to reinterpret her story of failure for losing her child. She suffered greatly from highly problematic parenting, had limited modeling of effective and nurturing adults, and had been walked as a child from drug house to drug house (just as she had done with her son). Additionally, Luisa had to deal with violent relationships with boyfriends, her day-to-day motivation for life revolved around getting high — similar to many addicts — and she was only 16 years old. The totality of these facts barely dented the sense of failure that Luisa experienced regarding the loss of her son to Child Protective Services. In fact, even if we had recited a thousand times these explanations for why things turned out the way they had or we chanted the refrain, "you were doing the best you could" it would have had a limited effect on her interpretations and feelings about her son. Instead, Luisa benefited from a more spiritual approach that embraced that dramatic failure in her life.

## FORGIVENESS AND FAILURE

The fourth step in 12-step programs involves making a complete moral inventory of your life. The purpose of this step is to become completely honest about who you are and what you have done. At this point, there is no point in hiding, fooling yourself, or rationalizing. You realize that life right up to the present moment has unfolded as it has. You can decide to tell the truth about how your life has unfolded or you can focus on giving reasons for why things have happened. The "reasons" may form a good story about your life; however, they may also cloud the essential nature of your behavior and choices, and the arrived-at reasons may obscure the raw description of life occurrences.

The fourth step allows you to settle into the narrative of your life failures, as well as its successes and accomplishments. Participants bring their dark, inner secrets to light so that the world can face them as they are. A sponsor bears witness to the fourth step and in most treatment programs group members get to hear the person's stumblings and bumblings of the past. People at this point do not say, "Don't be so hard on yourself," nor do they say, "It is understandable that you behaved this way; perhaps you should focus on the strengths of what you did." Instead the person hears words like, "Thank-you" and absorbs looks of compassion from those in the room who have tasted failure in much the same way.

Luisa deals with the failure of losing her son in this kind of open way. She allows for me and her group members to love her for who she is — failure and all. She is honest with herself and no longer has to hide. She believes that God forgives her, though she is not quite ready to forgive herself. Luisa has taught me how powerful it may be for clients to hear our own self-disclosed stories of failure.

## Universality of Failure

Luisa says that as she sits in her transitional living program she sometimes feels bereft over her past mistakes. She is happy to be playing with her young daughter and is feeling relieved to move away from her mother and to establish a degree of independence. Although she experiences this kind of fulfillment and relishes the bond that she has with her daughter, the loss of her son haunts her. The good feelings and positive events of the day can be overcome by her sense of failure regarding the events related to having her son taken away.

Luisa said that *what really has helped her in these times is being aware of how I failed with my own child.* My failings as a father make her failings as a mother acceptable. She knows that my intentions were not to fail, she knows that I am a decent person, she knows that failure is a part of life, albeit a painful one. If I, as the practitioner, can face failure and declare to the world that I have done it, then maybe she is not such a "piece of shit" (to use her language) for experiencing her own failures.

This discussion is not a treatise for excitedly telling people what failures they all are. It makes sense with some clients to have them disentangle their experiences. Clients who are quick to blame themselves for their sexual or physical victimization need to work from a base that removes shame and responsibility for what has occurred. The nuanced discussion of failure is not productive in these instances. As well, there are people who have successfully rewritten the story about their victimization that specifically excludes the concept of personal failure. This rewritten story has brought relief and often should not be compromised.

The emphasis here is to come to terms with failure in your own life so that you are prepared to help your clients face it in theirs. As Natalie Goldberg (2004) wrote in her Introduction to the book *The Great Failure*, "I wanted to learn the truth, to become whole. I wrote this book in the hope of meeting what's real. It is my humble effort to illuminate the path of honesty" (p.3). When we are honest about our own lives, we see that we have experienced failure in our relationships, our family lives, our money matters, and in how we take care of our bodies. Some of us have alcohol and drug problems, gambling problems, infidelity, out-of-control teenagers, personal insecurities, depression, inflated egos, and family scandals. We face our shortcomings and the failures that may or may not be linked, and we bring compassion to ourselves. In this way, we are able to be present for our clients when they are facing similar situations. Because we have walked this path, we are able to help them face their own failures.

## FAILURES IN LIFE VERSUS MY LIFE AS A FAILURE

Joan Halifax's evening of failure did not mean that she was a failure. Our behaviors, actions, approaches, and choices may have led to disasters; however, we are still individuals worthy of love. We ourselves are not failures. Although some people have multiple experiences with failing and may conclude that the term *failure* describes who they are, we learn to embrace failure in such a manner that it does not take become our identity. We apply mindfulness to those times when we feel insecure or inadequate and we notice our fight-or-flight inclinations. We decide to face how unskillfully we communicated with our supervisor the other day or how the DUI we had last month is, perhaps, part of a bigger issue. Neither these issues nor more severe occurrences lead to the portrayal of the self as a failure. We learn to make this distinction for ourselves, and this process assists us in helping clients make similar distinctions.

### Acknowledging Failure as We Proceed

Our sessions with clients provide opportunities for many micro-failures. We sit quietly with a client but she wants us to say something meaningful and our minds have not yet formulated anything meaningful. We sense the failure within this particular moment that includes an unmet client need as well as our inability to even approximate meeting that need. We radically accept our insufficiency in this moment and, in a state of calm, let our thoughts come together in order for us to move forward. Maybe the best we can do during this time is to say, "I'm not really sure what to say right now," or "I need to think more about what you are talking about because I want to be able to help you and be useful." Maybe this moment of failure will transform itself and lead us to ask a question that explores a useful area related to the discussion. Maybe if we relax with our breath, we will find a direction that may bear fruit.

As we move ahead, there may be some larger mistakes that we make. Carolyn Dillon (2003) has written a whole book on errors in clinical practice. Sometimes these mistakes contribute to a rift that may occur between our clients and us. The term *empathic failures* captures the essence of some of these rifts:

> *Empathic failures* occur when clinicians miss the boat and reflect the wrong content, feeling, or meaning. At other times, we may drift from the moment and miss a very important theme or feeling altogether, all the while appearing to listen and nod attentively. . . .

Another empathic mistake interviewers sometimes make is to confuse one client's story for another's and make a remark about an event or loved one unrelated to the client, hurting the client's feelings. The client may think, "I'm indistinguishable from all the others." (Murphy & Dillon, 2008, p. 142)

Our first step in dealing with failures—however large or small—is to acknowledge them. As we become more comfortable with failure being a consistent thread, we are able to face it with equanimity and clarity. With some of the bigger issues, we acknowledge to ourselves the sense that "something didn't go right," or "she seemed to walk away from this interaction dissatisfied," or "I should have handled that differently," or "my irritation with my client was unfair to him; I was in a bad mood and I treated him unfairly."

To complete our task in dealing with failure, we decide whether it would be helpful to patch up some of the difficulties. There may be instances where it makes sense to leave the dirt under the rug. We do not want to stir people up just so we feel good about ourselves for addressing the messes that we made. However, it makes sense many times to address our mistakes and failures. Initiating this process models honesty, comfort with failure, the capacity to address problems, and the caring and commitment to "get it right." Additionally, revisiting failures may change around the client's perception of the entire helping experience. Rather than interpreting our actions as indicators of noncaring or insensitivity, there is an opportunity to "right the ship" and keep the relationship on course.

Righting the ship may occur in our here-and-now interactions with clients and colleagues. As we tune into people's reactions, we notice their distress (or perhaps what we interpret as distress) and we take account of it. We become inquisitive, uncomfortable, confused, or compassionate about what had just happened. We tell ourselves, "let's stop" and we cultivate the intention to process and explore what has occurred. We enter into the moment despite not knowing what our explorations will uncover. We open ourselves to the possibility that we may have failed and we welcome the dialog that ensues.

Sometimes, we are not quick enough or we were too conflicted to handle ambiguity and distress in the here-and-now. We often have the opportunity to retrace our steps and look at what occurred even if some time has already passed.

## Admitting Failure and Trying Again

I consistently encourage practitioners to revisit with clients events that occurred in prior sessions. In one instance, a client tentatively mentioned that "he thought he may be gay" and the client received a detached clinical response on the lines of "what was it like to share that with me." This kind of response was in accord with the kind of training that this clinician received. In a subsequent group with the same practitioner, the client mentioned that perhaps he would be better off with a different practitioner because of the practitioner's age.

We examined these interactions and tried to imagine what the client may have been looking for when he first tentatively mentioned that he may be gay. I examined the practitioner's beliefs and attitudes toward gays and lesbians and realized that he missed an opportunity to show the client his complete acceptance of him and his willingness to celebrate him for whom he was. In effect, the practitioner likely failed the client's test of him and his unstated question: "Is this *the* person who is going to be my ally and be truly comfortable, supportive, and accepting of me?" Because I consistently normalize our failures during our supervision sessions, the practitioner had little to hide or be ashamed of. He did not spend wasted effort on berating himself or attempting to rationalize his behavior or show me that he is, in fact, culturally competent across sexual orientations. We discussed how the practitioner could approach the client in a manner that he would address the client's concerns and how he would express his willingness to celebrate the client's journey and his sexuality. The practitioner did have this kind of conversation with his client and he and the client are now in a solid, mutual relationship, doing constructive work.

Sometimes facing our failures involves plunging ourselves into riskier waters than trying to solidify our relationships with clients. In some instances, I encourage workers and/or supervisors to apologize for one form or another of unskillful behavior with the intention of clearing new ground for an effective relationship. Apologies require courage in this litigious climate because they can be equated with wrong-doing and the person making the apology can, thus, feel more vulnerable. We let go of our fears and our stories about how dealing with failures will just make them worse, and we do the right thing for ourselves, our agencies, and our clients. This approach is a guideline for action; however, some individuals or agency cultures will exploit our honesty and vulnerability, so we do need to assess the level of risk as well as the potential reward. The risks associated with not addressing ongoing difficulties or not facing or expressing dissatisfactions are important to incorporate in the risk-reward equation.

Our failures that involve larger groups of people may be difficult to revisit. I was teaching a class one time when a racially charged remark was made that offended some of the students. As the remark rolled from the student's lips,

I froze (right between fight-or-flight). I was not totally sure what I had heard, but I felt offended and knew that others would feel particularly offended. I also felt protective of the Caucasian student who made the remark, because I sensed it was from ignorance rather than from a hateful intent. One African American student spoke in a fairly indirect way about what had just happened, not being sure (as I later found out) that we as a class could handle this kind of discussion. After the class, this same student approached me, and I apologized to her for failing to address what had happened.

In a subsequent class, I prepared those in attendance for a discussion. I mentioned the difficulties of these discussions—they contain elements of fear, ignorance, confusion, and sometimes hatred. I was not removed from these elements in that my own fear, confusion, and denial contributed to not dealing with what had occurred at the time that the comments were made. We were to engage in the conversation as a group in order to understand what had happened and to learn about the sources of the feelings, thoughts, and behaviors of people in the class. I encouraged people that, though they may be angry with my failing to address this matter in the moment it happened, to consider accepting my present intention to build understanding.

I believe that taking ownership of my own failures gave permission for others to honestly explore the dynamics of the issues and to accept the shortcomings of our fellow class members. Various students commented later about the positive nature of the class discussion that emerged. This sentiment occurred despite the offending student's never fully dropping her defended posture.

It may seem like *accepting failure* paves the way for continued failure and lowers the bar of expectations. Many football coaches, for example, will say things like "failure is unacceptable"—with the notion that such talk motivates players to push toward victory. Some athletes, themselves, will say that their fear of failure drives them to succeed. I think that there are two issues regarding the acceptance of failure. First, the process that clients go through—moving from pain and difficulty to change and health is not necessarily comparable to winning a football game. As discussed earlier, change takes root in an environment of acceptance of what is. We "get real" about what has happened and how we are living. We face our secrets and bump into barriers along the way. We face our failures, but not so we can continue to repeat them. We face them precisely so that we can learn from them and move beyond them. Imagine, for example, if as a country we had honestly and completely faced the depth of pain and failure of our actions in Vietnam. Imagine how this act of collective courage would have affected the kinds of decisions that have been made since then.

Second, the acceptance of failure does not equate with apathy toward clients nor does it mean that we do not care about whether they succeed or fail. Our intention is to help. We do our best in this regard; however, we know that small and large failures are sometimes on the horizon. We are prepared to work with those failures as they arise and do not indulge ourselves in becoming despondent or despairing. We know that failure is a part of this ballgame, and we do not quit on our clients or seek to write them off with demeaning labels when things do not turn out as we would like them to.

## LABELING TO REDUCE FAILURE

What internal benefits accrue from applying pathologizing labels to clients? In my discussions with colleagues, one benefit becomes obvious. As we diagnose clients, particularly with personality disorders, we create a pathway to avoid feelings of failure. The authentic suffering of the individual as well as our limited ability to help is wrapped up into a neat package with the label "borderline personality disorder" or "narcissistic personality disorder." As a result, the practitioner's sense of failure for limited progress is diminished. I have experienced a degree of relief when contemplating these labels because the socially constructed personality disorders seem to contain a story that the clients who "have them" are a difficult bunch.

Embracing failure is an antidote to embracing labels that are dismissive and that—in some people's minds—may minimize practitioner responsibility for effective work. As we face failure, we contend with the reality that to some degree we are together sharing a life that contains pain, unskillful behavior, and sporadic and unpredictable gains. We and our client may both suffer through times when we feel incompetent and lost, and through times when we wonder whether anything good can come out of the helping relationship.

## FAILURE AND A NEW BEGINNING

We learn to embrace the "full catastrophe" of life, as John Kabat-Zinn (1990) says. The full catastrophe includes our failures as well as well as the richness, enormity, impermanence, unpredictability, chaos, sorrow, richness, and joy inherent in the human condition. With mindfulness, we learn to "see each moment as a new beginning, a new opportunity to start over, to reconnect" (p. 19).

Therefore failure, in effect, summarizes a series of events that occurred in the distant or not so distant past. We relax into our story about failure so that ultimately we can forgive ourselves, cool the flames of nonacceptance and denial, and move to the present moment where we live the "new beginning." We face failure and deal with it so that we will be able to embrace the full catastrophe. We realize that the one who embraces the full catastrophe

> embodies a supreme appreciation for the richness of life and the inevitability of all its dilemmas, sorrows, tragedies, and ironies. His way is to "dance" in the gale of the full catastrophe, to celebrate life, to laugh with it and at himself, even in the face of personal failure and defeat. (Kabat-Zinn, 1990, p. 5)

We confess and live with our failures and move forward in life realizing that more failure awaits us. As we are increasingly able to maintain a compassionate smile and look failure in the eye, we cultivate qualities that will help our warrior's journey upstream.

# Chapter Ten

# SWIMMING UPSTREAM WITH A WARRIOR'S HEART

*Beyond Working a Human Services Job*

*To take one step is courageous;*
*to stay on the path day after day,*
*choosing the unknown, and facing*
*yet another fear, that is nothing*
*short of grace.*

—Danna Faulds

*Do not waste your time by night or day.*

—Zen Master Dogen

The term *warrior* may turn some of us off because it conjures up associations with the violent world in which we live. We may prefer the soft and nurturing language of acceptance, presence, bearing witness, and open-heartedness. In our preferences, we perhaps shy away from discussing what actually makes for a strong back.

We must face the reality that we often need to *swim upstream* (as Zen Master Joan Halifax often says) in order to realize the sacred path of helping others. As mentioned in Chapter 1, there are people who seek to reduce the helping endeavor to quantitative puzzles and who may have little patience for the spiritual perspectives advanced here. In addition to our swimming upstream as helpers, we also come face-to-face with our own medical, emotional, familial, and social challenges that test our resolve and our mettle. We therefore endeavor to cultivate the qualities that nourish the warrior's heart that is needed as we negotiate difficult waters.

A Zen journey of helping involves the development of the warrior's heart, and the Zen tradition incorporates a sharp edge that assists us in being present and telling the truth in the midst of a world filled with delusion and denial. In addition to our commitment to honesty, our swim requires a healthy dose of courage and humility. People sometimes do not want to hear our thoughts or touch our pain, so we need to be courageous if we are to press forward. Our courage permits us to speak even "as our voice is shaking."

We also need to be aware that we may alienate people with unique perspectives or approaches. It is easy to appear self-righteous and arrogant. We therefore confess that we do not know for sure and admit to our failures and shortcomings. Our humility makes apparent that we are "them," and enables us to be approachable and effective.

During a forum that focused on providing assistance to soldiers returning from Iraq, licensed therapist and Vietnam War veteran Ray Bacigalupi, MFT, embodied these qualities of honesty, courage, and humility as he took attendees on what he called his journey "In and Out of Armor." The helping practitioners bearing witness to Ray's narrative were visibly moved and inspired. Although each person's manifestation of the warrior's heart is unique, I wanted to share, with Ray's permission, his talk from the Therapist for Social Responsibility Forum.

## IN AND OUT OF ARMOR

A few years ago I gave a speech in which I invited the audience on my journey that I called "In and Out of the War Zone." Today, I invite you to accompany me on a continuation of that journey that I am calling "In and Out of Armor."

My personal traumas, provoked by my family of origin, the school system, and cruel children led me to create an armor that allowed me to disconnect in order to survive. My Vietnam experience reinforced it. During my brief journey today, I will try and remove some of my armor as I share my thoughts and experiences with you.

I was 19 years old in 1966. Despite a traumatic childhood, I was completely unprepared for my military experience. First, there was the initial shock of being drafted and going through basic training. Then deployment to Vietnam in 1967.

There assigned to an army personnel carrier, I witnessed atrocities first hand.

- I witnessed an alcoholic sergeant order a private to chop the head off a dead Viet Cong soldier boy with a machete so he could keep the child's skull as a souvenir.
- I watched as a young girl's head was blown off.
- I witnessed local Vietnamese men carrying a pile of dead children in a blanket after a battle was fought in their village.
- I was there when U.S. military spotters gave the wrong coordinates to an army mortar unit and saw seven U.S. soldier boys killed and many seriously wounded.
- I watched as antipersonnel mines shot out 700 ball bearings that shattered bone and tore through flesh when they were detonated at us from the trees.

In 1968, my tour of duty in Vietnam ended when I was seriously wounded. After receiving the Purple Heart, I was honorably discharged.

When I returned from Vietnam, I was depressed and anxious. Fourth of July events and cars backfiring scared me. I found myself having recurrent nightmares of dying children or being captured by the enemy and tortured or being forced to return to Vietnam to serve again and again. The continuing controversy over the correctness of the war confused me.

When I was 22, I found my way to the VA's mental health clinic where no one asked about my experience in the military or treated me for PTSD. Medications I was given turned me into a zombie and I quickly discarded them. For the next decade, I self-medicated with alcohol and street drugs. I ignored politics and world events, kept relationships superficial, and

*(Continued)*

avoided commitment. I withdrew within myself, in my familiar armor, although underneath I was desperately needing connection.

I slowly but gradually risked enough to become a husband and a step-dad to young children. I did the work necessary to become a therapist. My life wasn't perfect but it worked well and my armor was unnecessary as long as I didn't venture too far out of my limited world.

Then in 1991, the first Gulf War triggered some anxiety and depression. I quickly re-armored and blocked out world issues.

But 10 years later, 9/11 and the invasion of Afghanistan started flooding me. By 2003, the shock and awe of our preemptive attack on Iraq broke through my armor and shocked and awed me into tears, confusion, anxiety, and rage. My limited world of being a loving husband, stepdad, and compassionate therapist wasn't enough anymore.

For the past 4 years, I have partially returned to 1967 and the horrors of Vietnam. I find myself having anxious feelings about life in general, nightmares, hopelessness, fear, anger, and disconnection. I have a strong desire to avoid, deny, and hide, to armor myself.

With the armor in place, I don't have to concern myself with the 30,000 children under age 5 who die everyday from hunger, thirst, and preventable disease; the children as young as 7 years old in third-world countries who are routinely sold into sex slavery; the billions of humans who live on less than a dollar a day; the political, military, corporate, and media lies, racism, genocide, greed, and cruelty; pollution of the world's natural resources; and needless wars.

These are some of the things I do not want to think of and don't when my armor is in place. There is a lot more I do not want to consider and even more I do not want to find out about.

When I take off my armor, I feel like a sponge that cannot hold one more drop. Others have called this compassionate burnout. When I am in this state, I call it survival. The constant bombardment overwhelms, confuses, and depresses me. Often, I just want to curl up in a fetal position and cry. I want to hide. That is when it is not making me furious and out of control. Then I want to explode and hurt someone.

At the same time, it is unacceptable to me to disconnect or hurt others. I want to be compassionate and more supportive—much less armored. It is difficult to stay in this space for long. Even now it is more of a place that I visit with my home being my armor.

As a therapist who helps others cope with difficulties and struggles, I know that to get through this I have to remove enough armor to connect and take action without becoming overly traumatized. Even if I had never been in a war zone, this would be a formidable task.

Some of the ways I have been keeping down my level of trauma while trying to help myself and others have been:

- Practicing staying in the moment.
- Associating with people who share similar values.
- Letting others know I need nurturing and then allowing them to nurture me.
- Taking positive action to help others.
- Staying connected when I most want to hide behind my armor.
- Sharing my feelings, thoughts, and visions; risking.

I'm not very good at it yet but I am practicing. A moment here, an event there. Such as today, sharing myself with you.

I have a particular perspective on war that led me to help found Therapists for Social Responsibility that recognizes the impact of politics on us personally and therefore advocates for values such as nonviolence, integrity, sustainability, and justice. I want to help vets, their families, and others while at the same time not be complicit with the culture of war and greed we are living in.

I am shocked at how desensitized we have become to atrocities of all kinds and concerned about what that means for our future. I am also disturbed by our society's ability to deny, avoid, and minimize the impact of war on the boys and girls who fight them. I just had nightmares of being forced to return to combat. Today, our soldiers have to return in reality.

Current military statistics suggest that fewer than 20% of our soldiers coming back from Afghanistan and Iraq have PTSD.

*(Continued)*

I believe that number is significantly underreported. If vets don't meet the criteria for PTSD, they are not counted even if they have significant problems related to their combat experience. Also, many soldiers see mental stress as a sign of weakness and are reluctant to admit the extent of their pain. Beyond this, a recent investigation found that military psychiatrists have been intentionally misdiagnosing soldiers with a preexisting personality disorder, a diagnosis that strips them of their medical and mental health benefits. The military doesn't provide the resources to treat those soldiers diagnosed with PTSD let alone those who don't make it into the health care system.

Additionally, there is a mental health crisis in the making worldwide. The Association of Iraqi Psychologists reported in January 2007 that of 2,000 people interviewed throughout Iraq, 92% said they feared being killed in an explosion. Sixty percent said the level of violence had caused them to have panic attacks and this prevented them from going outside.

Now the citizens of Iran are faced with the threat that the United States may at any time launch a preemptive war against them, possibly using nuclear weapons. And other countries are under siege.

Finally, how are we, as citizens of the United States, handling the constant background noise of war and injustice, knowing that it is our government using our tax dollars to kill and wound innocent civilians in other countries as well as our own soldiers? Are we experiencing our own form of PTSD? Are we disconnecting and putting on our armor when we can and feeling depressed and anxious when we can't?

I know I am. The most effective treatment for me has been to take small but persistent steps toward positive change while helping others on their path. If you are also concerned, I hope you will continue to participate in the work for peace and justice.

Thank you for sharing my journey In and Out of Armor.

Ray Bacigalupi, MA, MFT, is in private practice in Sacramento, CA, and a Vietnam veteran. He is one of the founding members of Therapists for Social Responsibility
www.therapistsforsocialresponsibility.org.

When we start with our traumas, insecurities, and failures, we let go of the armor that would prevent us from realizing the ultimate aim of Zen—to be aware and be intimate with *what is*. Telling the truth about our lives and embracing ourselves with an open heart is the antidote to our personal delusions and to the armor disconnecting us from others. We begin to make peace with our lives, and our stories about who we are and what we have experienced seem to loosen their grip on us. In spite of our wounds, we realize our inherent fearlessness to love the universe. We have prepared the ground for our Zen journey of helping.

## Liberation and Joy

We go into the darkness, we seek initiation, in order to know directly how the roots of all beings are tied together: how we are related to all things, how this relationship expresses itself in terms of interdependence, and finally how all phenomena abide within one another.

—Halifax, 1993, p. 137

As we shed our armor, we sense our connection with all beings around us. We deeply accept ourselves and others, which means we accept people who are different and who do not behave or believe as we think that they should. We relish the truth of uncertainty as well as unsolvable paradoxes such as maintaining boundaries in the midst of boundlessness or maintaining nonattachment in the midst of attachment.

We realize that letting go is paradoxically part of our swim upstream. We first let go of the delusion that we are in control. Although we may be willing to work hard enough to swim against the current, we swim with the realization that we do not have the final say regarding the outcome. We let go of the mind that obsesses about writing and rewriting the story of its own life and connect to the reality that there is no need to worship and attach to this individual "I." We bring ourselves fully to the present moment with our clients and sense that pure awareness governs the encounter. We gain glimpses of how the life that flows through these bodies "belongs" to no one, and we eventually let go of our attachment to our bodies and the stories of permanence that are associated with them. We face Ray Bacigalupi, and the wounded and traumatized participants of all wars and hardship with a heart and mind that has let go. We have not let go in the sense of becoming apathetic but in the sense of allowing a deeper purpose to guide us.

We swim upstream to find and realize our life's calling. We put aside convention that tells us to play it safe and make as much money as you can. We realize that our time is quite short and we decide how we will connect with our calling or deeper purpose and thus connect with the authentic truth of our lives, which transcends life and death.

One poignant story in this regard involves a famous tennis star Andrea Jaeger. Ms. Jaeger was a child protégé and by the time she was 16 was already one of the top tennis players in the world. During one year, she had been ranked as the number two female player. Despite all her success and money, it became apparent that tennis was not her calling. She, in fact, deliberately lost a Grand Slam final to Chris Evert because she knew that Evert cared more about winning than she did. Andrea took all her fame and fortune and opened a ranch in Colorado for children battling cancer. Many of them are dying. Her swim upstream is about living her deepest truth—what she describes as doing "God's work." A video that depicts her in action makes clear that she is no longer swimming upstream. She is able to listen to an internal voice that is stronger than societal pressures or externally generated fears (ESPN, 2007, http://broadband.espn.go.com/ivp/splash2?ceid =2929628).

Conceivably, we have already been called and we just don't know it. Perhaps some clarity about why we are doing this kind of work or what place this work has in our lives slightly eludes us. As helpers, we are fortunate. We somehow find ourselves involved with what is considered as venerable in all spiritual traditions—compassionately giving to others. We go on retreat, deeply contemplate, or pray about how we ended up here so that we participate fully in the day-to-day Zen of Helping, rather than just work at a human services job. As you sit with clients who suffer, they will sense how much of your effort is about executing a job or being connected to something noble or sacred, whatever form that takes.

Our open heart is a source of light and joy and, ultimately, feeds us as well as our clients. We reside in awareness and wonderment of the universe (or God), and we bring our spiritually nourished selves as we appreciate our day-to-day minutiae or a client's beautiful, subtle existence. We experience that there is one spiritual realm, home to the connection between our client's fate and the bigger picture, and in this wisdom we celebrate each moment. We project into the universe our sense of liberation and joy that—for even a brief moment—we have had the chance to live this human life. In our shared space, our clients begin to experience new possibilities.

Over time, we reside in the awareness that our clients have given us immeasurable gifts. Our strong back and soft front has become a major thread of our transformed lives, and without our clients, the tapestry would not have been the same. As they continue to watch us closely, our clients learn how special they are. In grace for all the contributions that our clients have made, we sit down with them and become part of each other's lives.

# BRIEF INTRODUCTION TO BUDDHISM AND ZEN

Zen's penchant to be nonconceptual, paradoxical, and downright mischievous means that it is difficult to summarize. Zen teachers and scholars (Ferguson, 2000; Loori, 2004; Merzel, 2003) often begin their discussions with comments such as:

> [T]he essence of Zen may be impossible to capture in words. . . .
> But when we speak about Zen, we need to remember that no matter
> what we say, it will miss the mark; it will be limited and insufficient,
> only one view of the whole. (Merzel, 2003, pp. 9–10)

One scholar (Ferguson, 2000) commented that even "[t]he word Zen itself . . . remains largely undefined" (p. 3).

Because Zen philosophy and practice is rooted in Buddhism, a brief discussion of Buddhist history and principles will help us make some sense of Zen. Some 2,500 years ago, Siddhartha Gautama led the protected life of nobility in a land that is now part of India. The most-often cited story is that Siddhartha's father was a king, and that Siddhartha's childhood displays of extraordinary intellectual, artistic, and physical gifts made him well suited to succeed his father's throne. Siddhartha though did not succumb to his father's plans for his life. He sensed that he needed to connect with the larger world outside the palace walls. When Siddhartha ventured out, he witnessed unimaginable suffering and was forever transformed. He realized that he had to choose between a life of delusion sequestered behind palace walls or a life in the larger world community, contributing to humanity's well-being.

185

The world behind walls in some ways is a metaphor for the walls of our mind that we construct. We feel aversion toward pain, difficult experiences, and people who do not think, act, or look like us. We conspire to avoid what we judge as unpleasant and we hold on, cling to, or crave what we judge to be pleasant. We try to protect ourselves through self-inflation, judgmentalism, and denial, or we sense that our walls have not kept us happy and we engage in self-hatred, denigration, or despair. It is delusional to believe that well-constructed walls will prevent suffering. Whether we are inside the palace or the small, craving, and aversive mind, we will eventually become sick and have pain. We will lose the people around us. These are difficulties that everyone in the world faces.

In our fearful and aversive small mind, we sense that if we venture outside, we will have to face a lot. Many times we make the strange decision to stay small and constricted, even though — in the long run — this strategy will not work. As I said, not only will we encounter common dilemmas (e.g., sickness and death), residing in our small mind nurtures the delusion that we are separate from other people. The delusion of separateness leads to faulty decisions in life — such as, it is okay to kill as long as I am not the one being killed.

Siddhartha sensed that the world of joy and ultimate truth lay in the larger world or what Genpo Merzel likes to call "Big Mind." He moved outside the walls of his deluded, constricted mind and attempted to meet reality. His first approach was to live an ascetic life and travel with others who were committed to a similar path. This path involved immersion into austere conditions for 6 years (Merzel, 2003). One such practice was eating one grain of rice daily over an extended period of time. From malnourishment and poor self-care, Siddhartha was near death. Fortunately, a villager found him barely alive and fed and clothed him.

Siddhartha realized that neither palace extravagance nor harsh austerities and self-induced suffering was the correct path for discovering the truth. He learned that he needed to travel the Middle Way between extremes. The Middle Way is not mushy centrism that we may associate with some politicians; it represents not getting attached to either side of an apparent duality. In this case, the duality was merging with suffering (the ascetic life) or avoiding suffering and engaging in indulgences (the palace life). Living the Middle Way means we do not argue for one over the other. Protection and suffering are intimately connected — two sides of the same coin. In the Middle Way, the Buddha took care of himself, protected himself from harm, and recognized that suffering would still visit. (The application of the Middle Way beyond dualities is covered in Chapter 7.)

While living the Middle Way, Siddhartha was strong enough to continue his mission of relieving humanity from suffering. He realized that he no longer had to strive and work so hard in order to realize deep understanding (Merzel, 2003). He vowed to sit under the Bodhi tree until he realized truths that would benefit all human beings. Because Buddhism is more focused on principles and teachings than events, there are different accounts of what happened at the time that the Siddhartha became enlightened. Some say the earth shook and animals celebrated, while other teachers talk about the "legend" or "story" of Siddhartha's enlightenment. After a short period of time in retreat, Siddhartha began to teach. His wisdom liberated many and his sheer presence and radiance was remarkable. Siddhartha engaged with the world with such vivid clarity that he was named Buddha, which means "the awakened one."

The Buddha delivered discourses for nearly 45 years, and the neurosciences, behavioral sciences, medicine, and healing arts are "discovering," studying, and applying his teachings 2,500 years later. (See Nhat Hanh, 1998, for an accessible overview of major teachings.) Buddhist teachings (also called dharma) were often transmitted through lists because they could be collectively retained and orally transmitted. The Four Noble Truths represents the most essential Buddhist teaching. The Noble Eightfold Path is intimately connected with the Four Noble Truths.

The First Noble Truth is that suffering exists. The Buddha stated that the main teaching throughout his life was suffering and the end of suffering. The Second Noble Truth is that there are causes of suffering. One fundamental cause of suffering is that we do not accept impermanence and that we fight against the reality of the way things are. As discussed in this book, Buddhism's emphasis on acceptance is not to be equated with in-action or complicity with injustice. Greed, hatred, and delusion (the Three Poisons) also cause suffering. The Third Noble Truth is the cessation of suffering. We can cultivate a spiritual approach that creates adverse conditions for suffering to take root. The cessation of suffering does not mean that suffering does not return. Suffering will arise but, with practice, it will not overwhelm us; we will be able to meet it with equanimity. The Fourth Noble Truth is that there are practices that make it more difficult for suffering to flourish. Living the Noble Eightfold Path generates joy, clarity, skillfulness, and mental concentration. An entire book by Surya Das (1998) amplifies the Eightfold Path principles that involve elements of behavior, ethics, clear understanding, and mental and emotional stability.

Evidence of Zen's origin dates to the second century some 600 years after the time of the Buddha. Zen teachings are usually traced back to Zen's introduction into China by Bodhidharma in the late fifth century, though scholars debate as to whether "writings attributed to Bodhidharma were actually written by him" (Ferguson, 2000, p. 3).

Zen myths, culture, and practice has focused on the bare bones of Buddhism — waking up in the present moment and becoming intimate with the world as it is. As we wake up and see reality clearly, we realize that there is nothing to attain or to strive for. We are already wonderful, enlightened beings, we are just so "asleep at the wheel" that we often do not realize our own fundamental nature.

We see clearly and become liberated when we become intimately connected to the present moment. Thus, Zen emphasizes metaphors and practices that enhance our affinity and our capacity for being present. For example, Kosho Uchiyama (2004), the head cook (tenzo) at a Japanese Zen monastery during World War II, discusses the supreme importance of the tenzo's work through a Zen Master Dogen (1200–1253) parable about Wu-Chao.

---

Wu-Chao was the tenzo or head cook of a monastery in the Wu-t'ai Mountains. One day while cooking, the Bodhisattva Manjushri appeared at the pot. Wu-Chao beat Manjushri to chase him from the kitchen. Wu-Chao exclaimed while striking Manjushri, "I would do the same to the Buddha himself if he appeared at the stove."

---

Being immersed in the present moment is of paramount importance, and the tenzo of a monastery becomes one with the task of cooking. Manjushri is a Bodhisattva — wholly committed to serving all beings — and should know better than to disrupt the sacred cultivation of Wu-Chao's concentrated mind. Manjushri's status within the monastery or his prior service in the world does not spare him of the harsh lesson meted out by Wu-Chao. Even the Buddha would get the same treatment.

What is striking about the story is how it stays with us. We could hear a lecture about how mindfulness is important, but it is more likely we will remember this story because of the themes we see within it and the way that these themes enter our consciousness. In Zen, nothing is more sacred than intimacy with the present moment. *The Buddha, himself, only points us to liberation, but liberation is realized through moment-to-moment practice.* If one becomes too enamored with the Buddha because of all he represents, then one is more likely to be in love with *ideas* about Buddhism than about actual liberation of self and all the world's beings. Neither the Buddha nor

Manjushri are beyond forgetfulness; if harshness eventually leads to the correction of their errors and to the world's liberation, then it is justifiable.

The *tenzo*'s story and my interpretations are not about justifying violence however. If your colleague knocks on your door and disturbs a session between you and a client, I do not advocate that you strike him or her. We need to cultivate the capacity to shift our focus and be present for whatever arises. The *tenzo*'s response was overly rigid. His field of attention could have expanded in order to include Manjushri, and his response could have been more skillful than striking him. Although difficult, the *tenzo* has to be with the meal, Manjushri's interruption, *and* his own thoughts and feelings regarding the interruption. He, in fact, was attached to an idea about the experience of cooking. The Zen of being with clients and providing help offers similar challenges.

The *tenzo* reflects Zen's orientation toward cultivating Samadhi or deep concentration. Merzel (2003) equates Samadhi with how artists or athletes will speak about "being in the zone." As levels of concentration deepen, petty thoughts, judgments, and worries melt away. The breath becomes the universe's breath, and life becomes the universe's life more than "my life." Although meditation and the enhancement of concentration may appear to be self-indulgent activities, the aim is to let the self "drop away," as Dogen says, and realize our inherent connection with all beings.

Joan Halifax consistently emphasizes that Zen is not a self-improvement program. Yes, there are benefits that one realizes, but its true aim is to face the truth of the world and to help all beings. In Zen, this is accomplished through becoming one with the present moment and responding skillfully to whatever arises. Unlike other Buddhist orientations that describe a prolonged individual journey (sometimes over several lifetimes) of progression, the highest forms of Zen practice and understanding can be realized now.

# REFERENCES

Anderson, H. (1997). *Conversation, language, and possibilities: A postmodern approach to therapy*. New York: Basic Books.

Asay, T. P., & Lambert, M. J. (1999). The empirical case for the common factors in therapy: Quantitative findings. In M. A. Hubble, B. L. Duncan, & S. D. Miller (Eds.), *The heart and soul of change: What works in therapy* (pp. 33–56). Washington, DC: American Psychological Association.

Austin, J. H. (1998). *Zen and the brain*. Cambridge, MA: MIT Press.

Battle, M. (1997). *Reconciliation: The Ubuntu theology of Desmond Tutu*. Cleveland, OH: Pilgrim Press.

Bein, A. (2003). The ethnographic perspective: A new look. In J. Anderson & R. W. Carter (Eds.), *Diversity perspectives for social work practice* (pp. 133–145). Boston: Pearson Education.

Brach, T. (2003). *Radical acceptance: Embracing your life with the heart of the Buddha*. New York: Bantam Press.

Brandon, D. (2000). *The Tao of survival: Spirituality in social care and counselling*. London: British Association of Social Workers.

Canda, E. R., & Furman, L. D. (1999). *Spiritual diversity in social work: The heart of helping*. New York: Free Press.

Canda, E. R., Nakashima, M., & Furman, L. D. (2004). Ethical considerations about spirituality in social work: Insights from a national qualitative survey. *Families in Society, 85*(1), 27–35.

Carson, C. (Ed.). (1998). *The autobiography of Martin Luther King, Jr*. New York: Warner Books.

Chodron, P. (1991). *The wisdom of no escape and the path of loving-kindness*. Boston: Shambhala.

Cohen, D. (2000). *Turning suffering inside out: A Zen approach to living with physical and emotional pain*. Boston: Shambhala.

Corrigan, P. W. (2007). How clinical diagnosis may exacerbate the stigma of mental illness. *Social Work, 52*(1), 31–39.

Das, S. (1998). *Awakening the Buddha within*. New York: Random House.

DeJong, P. D., & Berg, I. K. (2002). *Interviewing for solutions* (2nd ed.). Pacific Grove, CA: Brooks/Cole.

Dillon, C. (2003). *Learning from mistakes in clinical practice*. Pacific Grove, CA: Brooks/Cole.

Duncan, B. L., Miller, S. D., & Sparks, J. A. (2004). *The heroic client: A revolutionary way to improve effectiveness through client-directed, outcome-informed therapy.* San Francisco: Jossey-Bass.

ESPN. (2007). *Andrea Jaeger called to serve* [Video]. Retrieved July 13, 2007, from http://broadband.espn.go.com/ivp/splash2?ceid=2929628/).

Faulds, D. (2002). *Go in and in: Poems from the heart of yoga.* Greenville, VA: Peaceable Kingdom Books.

Ferguson, A. (2000). *Zen's Chinese cultural heritage: The masters and their teachings.* Boston: Wisdom.

Furman, R., Langer, C. L., & Anderson, D. K. (2006). The poet/practitioner: A new paradigm for the profession. *Journal of Sociology and Social Welfare, 33*(3), 29–50.

Gilbert, M. (2000). Spirituality in social work groups: Practitioners speak out. *Social Work with Groups, 22,* 67–84.

Glaser, A. (2005). *A call to compassion: Bringing Buddhist practices of the heart into the soul of psychology.* Berwick, ME: Nicolas-Hays.

Glassman, B. (1998). *Bearing witness: A Zen master's lessons in making peace.* New York: Bell Tower.

Goldberg, N. (2004). *The great failure: A bartender, a monk, and my unlikely path to truth.* New York: HarperCollins.

Green, J. W. (1999). *Cultural awareness in the human services: A multi-ethnic approach* (3rd ed.) Boston: Allyn & Bacon.

Halifax, J. (1993). *The fruitful darkness: Reconnecting with the body of the earth.* New York: HarperCollins.

Hayes, S. C., Follette, V. M., & Linehan, M. M. (Eds.). (2004). *Mindfulness and acceptance: Expanding the cognitive-behavioral tradition.* New York: Guilford Press.

Herman, J. (1997). *Trauma and recovery: The aftermath of violence—From domestic abuse to political terror.* New York: Basic Books.

Hodge, D. R. (2005). Spiritual ecograms: A new assessment instrument for identifying clients' strengths in space and across time. *Families in Society, 86*(2), 287–296.

Kabat-Zinn, J. (1990). *Full catastrophe living: Using the wisdom of your body and mind to face stress, pain, and illness.* New York: Dell.

Krill, D. F. (1978). *Existential social work.* New York: Free Press.

Krill, D. F. (1986). *The beat worker: Humanizing social work and psychotherapy practice.* Lanham, MD: University Press of America.

Krill, D. F. (1990). *Practice wisdom: A guide for the helping professional.* Newbury Park, CA: Sage.

Ladinsky, D. (Trans.). (1999). *The gift: Poems by Hafiz the great Sufi master.* New York: Penguin Group.

Linehan, M. M. (1993). *Skills training manual for treating borderline personality disorder.* New York: Guilford Press.

Linehan, M. M. (2003). *This one moment: Skills for everyday mindfulness* [Video]. New York: Behavioral Tech, LLC.

Loori, J. D. (Ed.). (2004). *The art of just sitting: Essential writings on the Zen practice of shikantaza*. Boston: Wisdom.

Malekoff, A. (2004). *Group work with adolescents: Principles and practice* (2nd ed.). New York: Guilford Press.

Martin, P. (1999). *The Zen path through depression*. New York: HarperCollins.

McNeill, T. (2006). Evidence based practice in an age of relativism: Toward a model for practice. *Social Work, 51*(2), 147–156.

Merzel, D. G. (2003). *The path of the human being: Zen teachings on the bodhisattva way*. Boston: Random House.

Miller, B. J. (1992). From silence to suicide: Measuring a mother's loss. In W. J. Blumenthal (Ed.), *Homophobia: How we all pay the price* (pp. 79–94). Boston: Beacon Press.

Mollica, R. F. (2006). *Healing invisible wounds: Paths to hope and recovery in a violent world*. Orlando, FL: Harcourt Books.

Murphy, B. C., & Dillon, C. (2008). *Interviewing in action in a multicultural world* (3rd ed.). Belmont, CA: Brooks/Cole, Thompson Learning.

Nhat Hanh, T. (1987). *The miracle of mindfulness: An introduction to the practice of meditation*. Boston: Beacon Press.

Nhat Hanh, T. (1993). *For a future to be possible: Commentaries on the Five Mindfulness Trainings*. Berkeley, CA: Parallax Press.

Nhat Hanh, T. (1995). *Zen keys: A guide to Zen practice*. New York: Three Leaves Press.

Nhat Hanh, T. (1998). *The heart of the Buddha's teaching: Transforming suffering into peace, joy, and liberation*. Berkeley, CA: Parallax Press.

Nhat Hanh, T. (1999). *Call me by my true names: The collected poems of Thich Nhat Hanh*. Berkeley, CA: Parallax Press.

Nhat Hanh, T. (2001). *Anger: Wisdom for cooling the flames*. New York: Berkeley Publishing Group.

Nhat Hanh, T. (2007). *The art of power*. New York: HarperCollins.

Rauner, D. M. (2000). *"They still pick me up when I fall": The role of caring in youth development and community life*. New York: Columbia University Press.

Remen, R. N. (2007). *The power of story* [CD]. Writers for Change Conference. San Francisco: VWTapes.

Rogers, C. R. (1961). *On becoming a person: A therapist's view of psychotherapy*. Boston: Houghton Mifflin.

Sahn, S. (1999). *Only don't know: Selected teaching letters of Zen Master Seung Sahn*. Boston: Shambhala.

Saleebey, D. (Ed.). (2006). *The strengths perspective in social work practice* (4th ed.). Boston: Pearson Allyn & Bacon.

Sanderson, C. (2003). *DBT at a glance*. Retrieved January 15, 2008, from www.behavioraltech.com/downloads/DBT_FAQ.pdf.

Schön, D. A. (1983). *The reflective practitioner: How professionals think in action*. New York: Basic Books.

Snyder, C. R., & Lopez, S. J. (2007). *Positive psychology: The scientific and practical explorations of human strengths*. Thousand Oaks, CA: Sage.

Suzuki, S. (1970). *Zen mind, beginner's mind: Informal talks on Zen meditation and practice*. New York: John Weatherhill.

Tanahashi, K., & Schneider, T. D. (Eds.). (1994). *Essential Zen*. Edison, NJ: Castle Books.

Tenowich, A. (2007). *Schizophrenia: Talking to God* [Video]. Retrieved October 18, 2007, from http://newsinitiative.org/story/2007/07/24/schizophrenia_talking_to_god/.

Uchiyama, K. (2004). The tenzo Kyokun and shikantaza. In J. D. Loori (Ed.), *The art of just sitting: Essential writings on the Zen practice of shikantaza* (pp. 55–62). Boston: Wisdom.

USA for Africa. (1985). *We are the world* [Video]. Retrieved July 15, 2007, from www.youtube.com/watch?v=WmxT21uFRwM/.

Wampold, B. E. (2001). *The great psychotherapy debate: Models, methods, and findings*. Hillsdale, NJ: Erlbaum.

Welwood, J. (1996). *Love and awakening: Discovering the sacred path of intimate relationship*. New York: HarperCollins.

Williams, M., Teasdale, J., Segal, Z., & Kabat-Zinn, J. (2007). *The mindful way through depression: Freeing yourself from chronic unhappiness*. New York: Guilford Press.

# INDEX

# ABOUT THE AUTHOR

Andrew Bein, PhD, LCSW, has 23 years of experience as a clinician, consultant trainer, and researcher. His rich work life includes the following settings: child welfare, public schools/special education, youth programs, multiservice centers, substance abuse, and private practice. Dr. Bein has served highly diverse communities and populations and has conducted over 80 national, state, and local presentations on a range of human service topics. Dr. Bein has been a Zen student for 10 years and is a Full Professor with the Division of Social Work at Sacramento State University.